Lose Wheat
Lose Weight

Lose Wheat
Lose Weight

**Antoinette Savill
and Dawn Hamilton Ph.D.**

Thorsons

Thorsons
An Imprint of HarperCollins*Publishers*
77–85 Fulham Palace Road
Hammersmith, London W6 8JB

The Thorsons website address is: www.thorsons.com
First published by Thorsons 2001

10 9 8 7 6 5 4 3 2 1

A catalogue record of this book is
available from the British Library

ISBN 978-0-0073-3092-8

Contents

chapter 1

The Start of a New, Healthy You

Do you frequently feel bloated, suffer from fluid retention or experience a general sense of sluggishness? Are you unable to lose those extra pounds, even though you are careful about what you eat? Do you sometimes feel that you've lost your sense of vitality and energy, and that life appears permanently grey? Are you confused about what to eat and what not to eat? If you have answered yes to any of these questions, this book can help. As the title suggests, it takes a close look at the relationship between wheat and weight loss, but that is only part of the story. In the chapters that follow, you will find advice and encouragement relating to every aspect of your daily diet.

What you will find here is not a diet based on calorie counting and fat units. There are no weight charts and no daily diet points to keep track of. In fact, I prefer to think of this programme not as 'a diet' at all, but instead as a move towards a new way of eating that is both highly pleasurable and extremely effective at enabling you to shed those extra pounds.

One of Life's Pleasures

Food can be one of the great pleasures of life but when we think about losing weight the last thing that normally springs to mind is pleasure. Instead we take it for granted that deriving any delight from food is denied us until our weight loss battle is over. And, for many people, a battle is exactly what attempting to lose weight turns out to be. We persevere with a calorie-counting diet for a few weeks, suffering a bland array of food until finally, out of utter despair and boredom, we throw in the towel and reach for a chocolate-chip cookie. And then, despite all our effort, discipline and hard work the weight often rebounds rapidly to its original level.

If, at the same time, we consider all the contradictory reports about food and nutrition that regularly appear in the media or in food manufacturers' advertisements, we find that the whole issue of what to eat or not to eat (both to lose weight and to be healthy) has become clouded with confusion. There seems to be little space left for food to be simply a source of pleasure and fun.

An Effective Eating Plan

What you will find within these pages is an eating plan that is both extremely effective at helping you to let go of those unwanted pounds and, at the same time, supportive of your overall health and well-being. Even better, this weight-loss plan actively encourages you to eat healthy foods that are tasty and pleasurable! It is time to say goodbye to the idea that in order to lose weight you have to endure boring and bland mealtimes. In this book there are plenty of ideas to tempt and tease your tastebuds and Antoinette's recipes should satisfy even the most discriminating of gourmet. Unlike many diets, this programme offers you a wide selection of foods to choose from, so you should never need to feel deprived. It is my firm belief that food can be simultaneously a pleasure, promote good health and encourage weight loss. And, provided that an individual is otherwise in good health, permanent weight loss can be achieved without a struggle.

How It Works

This weight-loss plan draws on principles from the fields of modern science (including how metabolism functions), nutrition and naturopathy (healing with natural approaches). These principles are outlined in the early chapters to explain precisely what does and does not work when it comes to losing weight. The later chapters provide all the practical information you need to put this programme into action.

No More Dieting!

The word 'diet' conjures up a host of associations for me and none of them are pleasant! It makes me think of deprivation, feeling hungry all the time, the need to have a monumental willpower and the boredom and effort of counting calories or fat units every day. I recall my previous attempts at calorie-reducing or fat-avoiding diets as periods of feeling physically exhausted, mentally sluggish and emotionally anxious. The whole process seemed like a constant struggle between my willpower and hunger pangs. Even worse, I can remember all the feelings of guilt and inadequacy, not to mention the sense of failure, that surfaced when I failed to achieve the weight loss I desired or whenever my willpower took a tumble.

I felt that there had to be a better way to achieve successful and permanent weight loss. What I have discovered is that this 'better way' is actually quite simple. It can be found by working in harmony with, rather than battling against, the body. When it comes to weight issues, we sometimes seem to view the body as some sort of traitor. We feel let down that it has managed to gain all those extra pounds so we go into battle against it by whipping up our willpower and restricting our food intake. We expect the treacherous body to put up the white flag immediately and surrender to our demand for instantaneous weight loss. Usually, however, the body has different ideas.

Calorie counting or adding up fat units, as most of us are painfully aware, seldom give lasting results. The reason is that these approaches fail to take account of many of the basic processes that govern the way the body uses energy and burns up fat. In other words, we are attempting to force the body into behaving how we think it should, but failing to give it the right conditions for meeting these demands.

A Strategy for Success

There is an alternative way, which is to adopt a weight-loss strategy that creates a powerful team between you and your body. That is the approach that you will find here. Working with your body, rather than struggling against it, makes weight loss a much simpler and more effective process.

The body is incredibly efficient when it comes to promoting health and vitality. It constantly strives to achieve balance and optimum health. To help it do its job properly, all we need to do is provide the right set of conditions. With these in place, and provided there are no underlying states of disease, weight loss can happen easily and effortlessly. It is also possible to lose weight while simultaneously supporting our body to move towards achieving better health. In fact, diet regimes that don't take the issue of overall health and well-being into account will always be less than successful.

Your Weight Loss Team

On this programme you are going to be collaborating with your body as a team. This team will include a selection of star players: modern science, naturopathy and optimum nutrition. These are powerful friends that will help you in a number of crucial ways. The information they offer will enable you to choose food that will enhance, rather than disrupt, the bodily processes that are involved in weight loss. They will provide your body with grade-A nutrients to ensure that these processes function efficiently. With their help you will achieve high levels of vitality and energy that will support your overall sense of well-being. In addition, these star players will show you a guaranteed way to end food cravings once and for all.

Team Players We Don't Need

What you don't want on your team are foods that can disrupt or actively sabotage your weight-loss efforts. Wheat, as is discussed at great length in Chapter Three, can be such a food. Many overweight people who follow a wheat-free diet for health reasons, (for example, to ease digestive complaints) find that they lose weight, even though they are consuming approximately the same number of calories as before. Removing wheat from the diet also frequently proves to be the solution for people who have been unable to get rid of bloating or fluid retention, despite being really disciplined in avoiding high-sugar and high-fat foods.

Although following a wheat-free diet is a key component of this programme, it is by no means the whole package. Other foods can also be very poor team players when it comes to weight loss. You will read about these foods in the chapters that follow. It is possible – and preferable – to select foods that will encourage the body to lose weight. Some of these choices may seem surprising. When we are trying to lose weight, we generally avoid foods that are high in fat because fat is high in calories. However, the issue of dietary fat and how this affects our ability to lose weight is more complex than a mere matter of calorie intake. Some fats actually help us lose weight, while others simply sabotage us, and some of the fats we tend to think of as good actually prove to be the worst offenders (Chapter Eight discusses dietary fats in depth).

The Quick-fix Doesn't Work

There are no quick-fix answers to successful weight loss. Following something like a calorie-counting diet for a few weeks and then returning to our old way of eating doesn't really get us anywhere. All that happens is that we feel frustrated and a failure because the weight has returned with a vengeance. Instead, the answer lies in reformulating our relationship with food. By making some small changes to the way we eat and live we can create a gentle and progressive shift towards healthier eating habits for life. This can provide us with a great deal of additional benefits beyond shedding those extra pounds. We may, for example, start to experience a sense of liveliness and vitality that we haven't felt for years. We may also find that eating no longer makes us feel highly tense and anxious, but is instead a nurturing and pleasurable experience.

Three Steps to Success

For a weight loss programme to be effective it should have three important components. It should ensure that the speed at which we lose weight is reasonably paced so that we do not shed vital muscle along with fat tissue. The weight loss should be permanent, so that it is easy to remain at our desired weight in the long-term. Finally, the foods that we do eat on our weight-loss plan should provide us with high levels of nutrients, so that we remain healthy and energetic during the process and after. There is no quick-fix single strategy that can fulfil all these conditions. To create the optimum conditions that your body needs if you are to lose those extra pounds healthily and permanently you need to combine several different factors. Each of these will be introduced in the chapters that follow.

Proof of the Pudding

As the result of applying the principles of optimum nutrition to my own life I know that these combined factors can definitely produce results. I no longer struggle with my weight or worry about how much food I am eating. The stress has been lifted from my shoulders, and letting go of the notion of calorie-counting and dieting has made my life easier and more fun.

Lynne is a good-looking and extroverted 56 year old. When I met her, she had been trying to lose weight for three years. It had slowly increased to 65.8kg/145lb but she felt her ideal weight was closer to 56.8kg/125lb. She had tried every type of weight-loss diet, from straightforward calorie counting, to avoiding fat, to a high protein-low carbohydrate plan, but all to no avail. Her weight stubbornly refused to budge. She came to see me principally for nutritional support because she lacked energy and had aches and pains in her joints. From an analysis of her symptoms, diet and profile I suspected that she might have a problem with eating wheat, so I recommended that she follow a wheat-free diet. I designed an eating plan for her that contained a healthy mix of proteins, carbohydrates and fats and made sure that all of the recommended foods contained adequate levels of vitamins and minerals.

Within a couple of weeks on the wheat-free diet Lynne noticed that her excess pounds were finally starting to shift. She stayed on the wheat-free diet for about two months, by which time all the excess weight had been shed. She bounced into my clinic and said: 'I am delighted to tell you that although my aches and pains have not entirely gone, I have lost over 20lb (9kg) in weight. What's more, I have not found the diet hard and I am not hungry all the time.' She also reported that she felt much more energetic and that the frequent bloated feeling and digestive problems that she had experienced for years had all disappeared. What had surprised her the most, though, was how easy it was to follow the programme. Lynne's weight remained stable in the long-term even though she later enjoyed an occasional meal that contained wheat.

Commitment Without Struggle

The early stages of following a wheat-free diet, plus adjusting to the other dietary changes outlined in this book, will require a degree of commitment on your part. However, as Lynne's experience shows, what you will not have to endure is the struggle, suffering and excessive effort that are generally associated with going on a diet. You can drop the 'no pain-no gain' mentality. It *is* possible to achieve effective weight loss without ever feeling hungry and without experiencing the host of uncomfortable side effects that usually go hand-in-hand with dieting.

In fact, as you will see, feeling really hungry is something you will actively avoid on this plan. And because you will never feel really hungry you won't need a will of steel to achieve the weight loss you desire. The approach that is outlined here revolves around creating a menu-plan based on healthy and nutritious foods, which should be a pleasure, not a struggle, to eat. Within a short period of starting to follow these eating guidelines you can expect to notice improvements in the way you are feeling and your overall sense of well-being. This will naturally give you the motivation and momentum to follow it through.

A Few Words on Food Intolerance

In Lynne's case one of the reasons that she was finding it impossible to lose weight was because she had an intolerance to wheat. Food intolerance is not the same as a food allergy (the difference between the two is explained fully in Chapter Three). Food intolerance has been found to be related to a range of physical complaints, but it is a condition that is very difficult to pin down because the symptoms seldom occur straight after the culprit food is eaten.

Intolerance can play an important role in weight loss. When somebody who is otherwise in good health – and who is eating a relatively healthy diet – has great difficulty in losing weight, it could be that food intolerance is playing a part. When this condition is present it also predisposes the body to hold onto excess weight and fluid. When the offending food is removed from the diet the body can re-balance itself and create the conditions for weight loss to occur.

Wheat and Weight Loss

Any food has the potential to cause an intolerance problem. But the majority of problems prove to be related to only a handful of different foods. The main culprit when there is an inability to lose weight is wheat. The whole of Chapter Three is devoted to the topic of wheat intolerance. It includes a self-test questionnaire so that you can assess whether this may affect you. Intolerance to one or a group of foods does appear to affect quite a few people. There are, however, plenty of people who can eat all types of food without experiencing any problems linked to intolerance.

Achieving an Ideal Weight for You

In this book you won't find any charts telling you what your ideal weight should be, based on criteria such as your height and build. If you've been on diets before, you probably know these charts off by heart anyway. What is more important, I believe, is that the only person who can define your ideal weight is you. You are an individual, not a statistic on a chart. Each of us has a unique biochemistry which influences which food, vitamins and minerals we need, and governs the level of activity required to maintain our well-being. It is important to start to tune into what our own bodies are saying regarding our individual needs. Once we have made this connection, we will find that the body gives very clear signals regarding weight, all of which are tailored to your own personal circumstances.

Reading the Signals

What kind of signals should you look for to determine your ideal weight? Rather than having a precise figure in mind, it is worthwhile to think in terms of a small range of about 2kg/4.4lb. For example, your ideal weight range might be 57–59kg/126–130lb rather than just 57kg/126lb. One of the key pointers to determine whether you are within your ideal weight range is that you will normally have an abundant energy when you are there. Go below the optimum range by even a few pounds and you will start to feel drained and tired. Friends may ask you if you are feeling unwell, as you may begin to look slightly drawn. Go over your optimum range by a few pounds and you will probably start to feel sluggish. By paying attention to these subtle messages you should soon get a clear indication of the weight that is best for you. However, you are unlikely to pick up these signals until your weight is close to this ideal range. If you are currently 9kg/20lb or 14kg/30lb above your optimum weight, you will need to start moving towards what you think is your ideal weight and pay attention to the signals once you are nearly there. If you are still unsure as to what weight you should be, the best thing to do is to visit your doctor, who can give you some very good guidelines.

Scales and Body Shape

The weight that registers on the bathroom scales can sometimes be misleading. Muscle tissue is heavier than fat tissue. So when you start exercising as part of your weight-loss strategy, the scales may seem to suggest you are not shedding much weight. What is actually happening is that fat tissue is being swapped for (heavier) muscle tissue. Although your weight may not have changed significantly, your body will definitely have changed for the better. The bathroom scales don't always tell the whole story. You need to observe changes in your shape as well.

When you start to listen to your body's signals you may find that your perfect weight is slightly more than you had originally thought. This is okay. We are not all designed to be a size 6. Sometimes we get involved in endless dieting because we are convinced that only a certain dress size will make us happy. This is unproductive in the long term. We are all unique in terms of shape and size, so forcing our bodies to be something they are not makes no sense. What is really great about getting to our personal ideal range is that it usually corresponds with the weight at which we look our best as well, even if this is a dress size larger than we really think we ought to be. So, when it comes to feeling great and looking great, trust your body to provide you with the right signals.

Becoming Congruent

As a nutritionist and a psychologist I am very aware of the influence that our mind and emotions have on our eating patterns. This book is primarily concerned with the nutritional aspects of healthy weight loss, but I believe it would be incomplete if the important role of our psychological selves were not addressed. For this reason, I want to raise a few issues that can unwittingly disrupt our attempts to lose weight.

Each of us functions as a unified whole. The body, mind and emotions are not simply separate parts that interact with each other; they effectively create a cohesive unit, which is what defines each person as a unique individual. What we think and feel on a regular basis is reflected in the body. It appears in the way we hold ourselves, the way we move and the way in which our bodily processes function. The condition of our body also has a big impact on our emotional self and on how our mind functions. For example, if we do not provide the body with the right type of food or adequate physical activity we may experience this on a mental level as an inability to concentrate and on an emotional level as feeling down or depressed.

Multi-faceted Emotions

Both the mind and our emotions are multi-faceted and complex. There are layers and layers of thoughts and emotions that we can unravel. Imagine the most beautiful and intricately-cut diamond that ever existed. Now imagine that you can only observe one per cent of that diamond at any one time. Each time you have another look at the diamond you notice something different. Looking at the diamond is similar to understanding the complexity of your emotions and thoughts. We can spend a lifetime getting to know ourselves or a loved one and still find that there is more to learn, more to uncover. This is what makes life so rich and interesting.

However, there are times when certain aspects of ourselves can be in conflict. When these aspects are battling against each other it can be very difficult to achieve a particular goal as we will inadvertently sabotage our own progress. For example, many of my colleagues from nutrition school started to practise as soon as they graduated. It took me 18 months. Consciously I knew that I had the necessary knowledge to do this work and that it could have a profound impact on an individual's health, but I would also find myself thinking: 'What if I am unable to help anybody?'. Emotionally, I was excited at the prospect of working in this way but also quite anxious. Importantly, I couldn't picture myself in this role. It simply didn't feel right; what did feel right at that time was the career that I was currently pursuing.

This was a classic case of being in conflict. I was being pulled in different directions by these opposing thoughts and emotions. This situation may have continued indefinitely had the manager of a health clinic not telephoned to offer me the opportunity to work there. Despite my reservations, I knew that this was a good offer, so I went ahead. After a short time my internal conflicts were resolved. The new career path felt a natural part of me.

Lack of congruency can impact upon any area of our life, including our ability to reach our ideal weight. When we are congruent losing weight becomes a purely physical issue: provide the body with the right type of food and create the conditions that it needs and weight loss will happen. But if our thoughts are conflicting and/or our emotions are not congruent then, even with the right physical conditions, we may still find losing weight difficult.

Setting Goals

I've already mentioned that you don't need loads of willpower to follow this weight-loss programme. This is because the types of food you are encouraged to eat are ones that will help you to avoid any physical cravings. It is important, however, to make sure that on an emotional and mental level you are committed to your weight-loss goals. This type of commitment does not simply involve a mental decision; it encompasses the whole of your being.

The most powerful motivation for achieving weight loss comes from internal and 'moving towards' factors. Do you want to lose weight because your partner or friends have told you that this is a good idea? Or is it because *you* want to? Do you want to lose weight because you really can't stand how you look right now? Or do you accept how you are at this moment, but feel excited at the prospect of changing your shape? Doing something for yourself is much more likely to bring success than doing it because others expect it of you. Moving towards an exciting vision of the future ('I'm really looking forward to wearing that stunning dress') is much more motivating than trying to run away from what you perceive as unpleasant in the present ('I can't bear to look at myself in the mirror the way I am now').

Losing weight can be a struggle when we perceive ourselves as we currently are in a negative way. It can be quite hard to be motivated if we are continually criticising ourselves. Statements like 'I hate the way I look. I feel my body is really horrible and I will only be happy when I lose all this ugly fat' only serve to create a battle within ourselves because we are rejecting how we are at the present moment. We may stick to a diet for a few days and then reach for some chocolate because 'my horrible body is never going to look good anyway, so what's the point?'. Of course, negative self talk such as this in no way reflects the reality of the situation. We would never say such unkind things to our friends, but when it comes to ourselves we can be the harshest critic.

A Positive Attitude

A totally different attitude is 'I am really keen to feel more alive, fit and vibrant, but while I am working towards this goal I still love my body exactly as it is right now. After all, my body is doing quite a good job of supporting my health and well-being. There are lots of really good things about it at the moment. I really like my (arms, legs, eyes, – whatever is right for you) and I love how these parts show to the world the unique beauty that is me'. This is a *moving towards* statement that doesn't reject how things are at present. It will create congruency between your mind, emotions and body, meaning that there is no need to battle or fight in order to achieve your goal. Instead, you will be able to move forwards with ease and pleasure.

In the next chapter you will read about the set point. This is a physical mechanism that makes it difficult to move from a certain weight unless you work with your metabolism in the right way. I have observed that people also have a 'psychological set point'. This is the weight that your mind/body/emotions see as being normal: the weight that 'feels right'. Some people indulge in overeating due to psychological triggers at the end of a diet. These have the effect of making their weight return to its previous level, and occur because a state of congruency has not been achieved. It is possible that the lower weight felt unnatural, uncomfortable or even a little bit scary. So the impetus to regain weight is a desire to get rid of these unpleasant feelings. This doesn't happen consciously. Someone doesn't wake up one morning and say 'Right, I've achieved my weight-loss goal, but now it's time to put it all back on again, so let's go to the kitchen'. Instead, the motivation to regain weight comes from a deeper level of the individual. However, if you can reach a state of congruency at these deeper levels you will be able to maintain your new weight in the long-term.

Shifting the Psychological Set Point

A method of achieving this congruency and shifting the psychological set point is to really get a sense of how you will be at your ideal weight before you actually get there. This involves physical and emotional sensations, not just your rational thoughts. Merely thinking that it would be nice to be 9kg/20lb lighter doesn't produce a strong sense of motivation. If you can really get in touch with how you would feel – on an emotional, mental and physical level – at your ideal weight, it is much more likely that you will achieve your goal and stay there.

There is a simple exercise you can do to see whether you are congruent in this respect. Take a couple of deep breaths, close your eyes and go within yourself. Take a few seconds to notice any emotions and how your body currently feels (tense, relaxed, happy). Now think about how life will be when you are at your new weight. Conjure up some images and scenes as if you were watching a TV movie with yourself in the starring role. Become aware of what you are feeling as these mental scenes unfold. Are the emotions pleasant or is there a subtle sense of discomfort? Next, switch into physical sensations and focus on how your body feels. Can you get a physical sense of how your body will feel at your ideal weight? Pay attention to any thoughts that float through your mind during this process. These might be positive ('I'm really looking forward to achieving this') or not so positive ('I've tried this before and failed, so why should this time be different?').

If you noticed any uncomfortable emotions, limiting thoughts or found it difficult to feel the experience on a physical level you may not be totally congruent. In this case, try the exercise again with this variation. While continuing to breathe slowly and deeply see yourself in your mind's eye at your current weight. On the mental TV screen visualise yourself losing weight at a very slow rate. Start with making yourself just 1kg/2.2lb lighter than you are right now. If this feels okay, reduce your weight by another couple of pounds. Keep reducing until you reach the lowest weight where you still feel 100 per cent comfortable on an emotional, mental and physical level. Make this the weight you are going to aim for as the first goal of your weight-loss plan.

It doesn't matter if this is just 500g/1lb less than what you currently weigh. Once you achieve this goal the momentum will start to build and you will shed more weight as time goes on. If you want to lose quite a lot it can be very difficult to imagine the reality of being at such a different weight. Taking it slowly and breaking your goal down into 'bite-size chunks' will enable you to shift your psychological set point at a steady pace. It is rather like walking up a very steep hill. If you look at the top you may think you will never get there. But if you set yourself targets (such as just getting to the next tree) before you know it you will have achieved your goal. What you are creating is a series of targets that work on all levels of your being, not just with your rational thoughts. Try and spend five minutes every day practising this exercise. Only visualise yourself at the weight where you still feel congruent. Make a note of any feelings or thoughts that occur as you do this. You may get some personal insights. Some of these may be uncomfortable, but even these may shift naturally. Keep focussing on where you want to be in the future and reward yourself for each success as your actual weight starts to drop.

chapter 2

Lose Weight
Without Struggle

This chapter explores two somewhat different approaches to weight loss – the scientific route and the application of some of the knowledge gleaned from the field of naturopathy. (Naturopathy uses natural approaches (diet, cleansing, lifestyle) to support the body's rhythms and processes. These approaches shift the body towards greater strength and balance, which then allows powerful self-healing mechanisms to operate.) Both of these approaches regard calories as only a very small part of the weight loss equation. Science suggests that how well our metabolism functions is a key indicator of weight loss or weight gain. Our understanding of the delicate and intricate processes of metabolism has advanced a great deal during the past decade. These developments have shed light on the underlying reasons why simply cutting calories does not work very well as a weight-loss strategy. Specific foods have a big effect on metabolism, so this chapter outlines some key ways in which nutrition can help to support the metabolic process.

Naturopathy doesn't pay much attention to calories either, but for different reasons. Natural approaches to weight loss focus on creating the right set of conditions within the body. If any of these conditions are lacking, then, even if we cut calories, the excess weight is unlikely to budge.

I believe that both modern science and naturopathy can help us solve the weight-loss puzzle. Both viewpoints complement each other, so there is no conflict in taking the best from each of these different fields.

In doing so we place ourselves in a pretty strong position to finally let go of those extra pounds without struggle, and we are less likely to put the weight back on afterwards.

The Calorie Myth and the Set Point

It sounds like common sense to suggest that weight loss depends on reducing our calorie intake, but cutting calories frequently fails to bring us the results we desire. The calorie-counting approach treats calories in the same way as we treat money in our bank accounts. Make a large number of deposits and the weight balance goes up. Make fewer deposits, but carry on spending as before, and the weight balance drops. This sounds straightforward enough but the body doesn't always respond in the way we expect. This is because the body has extremely sophisticated mechanisms that govern our weight, which the calorie-counting view does not take into account.

The other day a friend told me that she had decided to stop putting sugar in her tea. She had read somewhere that this would make her lose 4.5kg/10lb in a year. While this sounds like an easy way to lose weight, it is unlikely to work, because it does not reflect how the body balances calorie intake and expenditure. Let's assume that this strategy did result in her losing that amount of weight in a year (which is unlikely). What happens in year two? Presumably because she is still having tea without sugar she will lose another 4.5kg/10lb. At that rate, in about twelve years she would vanish entirely! Obviously this will not happen, but what the example illustrates is that the 'bank account' approach does not fully explain the process of weight loss.

Take a moment to think of some of the people you know who are not on a diet. It doesn't matter whether they are slim or if they could do with losing a few pounds. When people are not dieting they generally spend absolutely no time thinking about calories. What this means is that calorie intake and expenditure naturally vary from day to day. One day might include lots of social activities so a large amount of food might be eaten. Another day might be crammed with appointments, leaving only enough time to grab a quick snack. Despite these fluctuations in calorie intake and expenditure, the weight of a person who is not on a diet will tend to remain pretty much constant. If calories alone were responsible for weight gain or loss, then everybody would experience weight fluctuations all the time because of the regular variation in calorie intakes. Why this usually doesn't happen is because the body has developed a very clever mechanism to keep weight pretty constant.

The Survival Mechanism

Survival is the most important priority for the body. Throughout history, the food supply has fluctuated due to bad weather, wars, plagues and crop failures. Our metabolic systems have adapted to cope with these frequent variations in food intake. This is very useful for surviving periods of food shortage, but when it comes to a deliberate attempt to lose weight things are a little more tricky. Calorie-counting often fails to result in permanent weight loss because progress is sabotaged by two metabolic processes.

The first of these is a sophisticated mechanism that can vary the speed at which energy is derived from food. It is particularly efficient at this job whenever calorie intake falls. We might lose a reasonable amount of weight (including some excess fluid) during the first couple of weeks of a calorie-restricted diet but then the progress seems to falter. What has happened is that the body has adapted to the restricted calorie intake and is using such calories as it does receive much more efficiently than before. It therefore no longer needs to burn off fat stores to meet the calorie deficit.

The second metabolic process is even more complex. This is a mechanism that is often referred to as the set point. It has one principal objective and that is to keep the body's weight at what it perceives to be 'normal'. For the body 'normal' is the weight it has been for the past few months. Whenever we drop a few pounds in a short period of time the set point mechanism kicks in because this divergence from 'normal' is perceived as a potential threat to our survival.

Shifting the Set Point

There are extremely effective methods for shifting the set point's 'weight thermostat' away from what it thinks of as 'normal' to the weight we would like it to be, but calorie counting is not one of them.

This is why. There are two types of hormone involved in appetite control and the effective storage of energy derived from food. One set of hormones signals the brain when it is time to eat and another hormone signals the brain that we're full. These same hormones instruct the body to shed energy (lose fat tissue) when we are full and conserve energy (store fat) when we are hungry. When we cut calories and lose a few pounds these appetite control hormones are adjusted dramatically. First, there is an increase in the level of hormones that send a signal to the brain telling us to eat. At the same time, the level of the 'I'm full' appetite hormone falls. This fluctuation in hormone levels also signals the body to hold onto energy (keep hold of fat tissue) as much as possible.

What this means is that while you know you are cutting calories in an attempt to lose weight, your body is working as hard as possible to hang on to every ounce of fat so that the set point can be maintained. Furthermore, in the face of the overwhelming power of chemical messages that are crying out 'eat, eat, eat!' is it any wonder that your willpower weakens and you give up your diet?

Seeking Stability

Varying the speed at which we use calories and adjusting our hormone levels are the body's way of maximising its efforts to rapidly replenish any weight that has been lost and return to 'normal' weight. The set point likes stability. It doesn't want our weight to move much from the level that it has been for the past six months or so. This works with weight increases, too. That is why we can eat high levels of calories for short periods and not gain weight. This mechanism also explains why people who are not dieting can regularly vary their calorie intake and remain at the same 'normal' weight.

About 90 per cent of people who follow a calorie-restricted diet regain all the weight they have lost within a short time. A further effect of a calorie-restricted diet is that any weight lost usually consists of both fat tissue and muscle tissue. Burning up fat tissue is good news but losing muscle tissue is not. As soon as we succumb to the chemical messengers' powerful entreaty to eat more food, what we digest is converted by the body straight into fat tissue. So after a failed low-calorie diet we may end up in a worse situation than when we started. Not only have we regained all the weight lost, but we now have more fat tissue and less of the important muscle tissue. This has a knock-on effect by reducing the efficiency of the metabolism so that it's harder to lose weight in the future.

Turning up the Heat

If simply reducing our daily calorie intake doesn't work because of the slowing down of our metabolic rate and the rebound to 'normal' weight, how do we reach our desired weight in a healthy and struggle-free way? The solution, is we need to work with, rather than against these physical processes.

Weight loss becomes much easier when we become more metabolically active. What this means is that we are effectively 'turning up the heat' of our energy-processing system at a biochemical level. Regular exercise, which needs to be both aerobic and strength-building, is one of the ways that we can improve the efficiency of the metabolism. This has little to do with the fact that exercise burns up calories. I always find the machines at the gym that tell me I have just used up 152 calories quite amusing for two reasons. First, using up calories isn't really the main benefit of exercise. And second, the machine seems very precise in determining how many calories were used (not 150 or 155, but exactly 152), which is nonsense, because it is unable to measure my unique metabolic function. What is important about exercising regularly is that it helps the metabolism to use up calories at a much faster rate in the long-term. Exercise also helps to build muscle tissue, which is more metabolically active than fat tissue.

Exercise is only part of the picture, however the type and quality of the food that we eat also has a significant impact on metabolism, so this eating plan is specifically designed to encourage the metabolism to work efficiently. By following a diet which provides you with all of the essential macro-nutrients (carbohydrate, protein and fat) in the right combination – and, most importantly, in the best possible form – you will find that weight loss becomes much easier.

The same eating guidelines are very good at dealing with cravings. You can forget the usual see-saw of feeling so hungry that you lapse into a binge. Managing cravings is such an important issue that the whole of Chapter Four is devoted to this topic.

All Calories are not Created Equal

Calories from different types of food have different effects on the body. A calorie derived from one type of carbohydrate food will support your metabolism and help you to lose weight. A calorie from another carbohydrate food can create metabolic havoc, which will disrupt your weight-loss efforts. Both give exactly the same reading on a calorie chart, but they act differently. The explanation is found in the way that the body processes these foods. Some carbohydrates are processed slowly, which helps to keep the metabolism functioning at an efficient pace. Other carbohydrates are processed very quickly, and confuse the metabolism. This process is explained in greater depth in Chapter Four as it is one of the key principles that will help you to overcome cravings.

All fat calories are not the same either. It is widely accepted that in order to lose weight we should cut down on fat because it is high in calories. But specific types of fat play a vital role in keeping the metabolism functioning healthily. When these fats are missing from the diet the metabolism can become sluggish and weight loss becomes harder than it needs to be. These particular fats also have a number of crucial functions to perform in keeping our bodies and minds in tip-top condition. So, while it is good to reduce our intake of 'bad' fats, your metabolism will work more efficiently if you have a small portion of healthy fats every day. Chapter Eight discusses the subject of fat in some detail, so you will know exactly which fats to eat and which to avoid.

Vitamins and Minerals

Metabolism is a very sophisticated process that requires a host of specific vitamins and minerals. These include many of the B vitamins, vitamin C, zinc and magnesium. If any of these are absent from the diet, the metabolism will not be operating at optimum efficiency. The foods that you are encouraged to eat on this plan are highly nutritious, so you should receive adequate intakes of these important nutrients.

This eating plan provides a healthy balance of carbohydrate, protein, healthy fats, vitamins and minerals. All of these need to be present in your diet if your metabolic system is going to work effectively. When the body receives the nutrition it needs it will start to shed excess fat tissue without the associated metabolic slowdown and burning of muscle tissue. What is more, the set point will not interpret the situation as 'famine time', so you will be able to shift your weight from what your body perceives as 'normal' to the new level you desire with permanent results and no rebound effects.

Fat, Fluid or Bloating?

Conditions such as fluid retention and bloating are extremely common. Excess weight may be a combination of both fat tissue and unnecessary fluid. Trying to combat the problem of excess fluid merely by going on a diet will not work. It is natural to drop some excess fluid during the first week or so of a diet, but after this point the surplus usually stays where it is.

Fluid retention is most obvious in the extremities of the body, such as feet, ankles, hands and face. But fluid can accumulate all over the body, including the abdomen, thighs, upper arms and buttocks. A simple way to test whether you are carrying excess fluid is to press your thumb firmly into an area of skin around your ankles or thighs. If the skin does not bounce back quickly and it appears 'springy' or 'spongy' this can indicate that fluid retention is present.

The body is about 70 per cent water. The brain is 85 per cent water and the muscles are 75 per cent. Even our teeth consist of 10 per cent water. This life-supporting substance is required by every single function of the body. There are a number of reasons why our fluid balance can be disrupted, but the most obvious cause is long-term dehydration. This doesn't mean that we are dehydrated to the point where we need to get urgent medical assistance. Instead, it is a long-term state where we regularly fail to give the body the amount of fluid it needs. Unless you can honestly say that you drink at least 1.5 litres/2½ pints/1½ quarts of water per day, every day, and that you seldom drink coffee, tea and cola, you are more than likely dehydrated.

Another way to assess whether you are drinking enough water is to check the colour of your urine. The darker it is, the more dehydrated you are. When you are taking in enough water your urine will be virtually clear.

Lack or Excess?

How is it possible to be dehydrated, yet suffer from water retention? Surely being dehydrated implies a lack, rather than an excess, of fluid? This seems logical but it is perfectly possible to drink too little to support bodily functions efficiently, while simultaneously storing excess fluid. The problem is stuck in our tissues, so cannot be accessed by the parts of the body that need it. And because we are dealing with a lack, rather than an excess, trying to relieve the symptoms of fluid retention with diuretics (water pills) will only make the situation worse in the long-term. Few people drink enough water to keep their systems functioning optimally and frequent use of cola, tea and coffee – including decaffeinated coffee – increases the likelihood of dehydration, as these drinks have strong diuretic effects on the body.

Dehydration can affect our ability to lose weight in other ways as well. When we have been in a state of partial dehydration for a long time (for many people, this means years) we may lose the connection with the body's signal for thirst. When this happens it is easy to confuse the signal for thirst with hunger. The body tells us it would like some water but, as we think we are hungry, we respond by eating. As we haven't given the body what it needs the thirst/'hunger' message is left on. In a roundabout fashion, dehydration can therefore cause us to overeat. The body's elimination channels (e.g. the digestive system, genito-urinary system and lymphatic system) all need an adequate intake of water if they are to function optimally. Weight loss is both easier and more effective when these elimination channels are working well (more on this later). Something as simple as drinking more water can have really powerful effects, helping you to get rid of excess fluid and to lose excess fat tissue as well. When you are dehydrated, drinking more water will also have a positive effect on your general well-being. The condition of your skin may improve and you are likely to have a lot more energy.

The Food Intolerance Factor

Food intolerance can also be implicated in fluid retention. The offending food appears to affect the body by increasing the permeability of the capillaries, which means that extra fluid flows into the cells. The most common culprit is wheat. Lynne, who we met in Chapter One, lost over 9kg/20lb in two months when she eliminated wheat from her diet. I would estimate that about half of this weight loss came about because of the removal of excess fluid from her body.

When food intolerance is a factor, even drinking lots of water will not totally clear fluid retention. The culprit food needs to be avoided for a period of time so that balance can be restored to the body.

Salt and refined sugar also have a role to play in this problem. A great deal of fluid is needed to metabolize foods that are high in refined sugar, so if we eat lots of these foods we will be holding a lot of water as well. Salt stops fluid from being removed from the body. Therefore, cutting down our salt and refined sugar intake is an important part of the strategy to alleviate fluid retention. Foods which can help to eliminate excess fluid include watermelon, celery and cucumber. Watermelon is excellent as a base for fruit smoothies (see Chapter Eight).

Abdominal bloating might be a symptom of fluid retention or it could be a sign that your digestive system is not dealing particularly well with a specific food. The most common food linked to bloating in the stomach area is wheat. As soon as wheat is removed from the diet this bloating can diminish rapidly, often within a couple of days.

Time for a Spring Clean

We need to keep our bodies clear of toxins and accumulated waste products if weight loss is to be effective and struggle-free. We accumulate waste from a whole range of different sources, including physical processes such as repairing cells (the dead cells need to be removed from the body). The body's elimination system consists of the liver, kidneys, lungs, digestive system, lymphatic system and skin. You will read a lot more about each of the individual parts of this system in Chapter Seven. It is definitely worthwhile making your body's elimination system one of the star players in your weight loss team. When we fail to support this system we can experience unnecessary side effects while losing weight and may well find it very difficult to shed excess pounds.

The waste products produced by the body spend a short time circulating through the bloodstream before being eliminated. Under normal circumstances these wastes are swiftly removed from the blood and discharged from the body. Sometimes, however, this process does not happen as efficiently as it should. This can occur when any part of the elimination system is not working at top speed, and the rate at which we get rid of unnecessary substances are removed from the body is slowed down.

Toxic Substances

Molecular waste is toxic and potentially damaging to the body, so it is not a good idea to have these substances circulating in the bloodstream. When they can't be eliminated from the body via the usual channels (perhaps because part of the system isn't functioning optimally) they still need to be taken out of the bloodstream as fast as possible. So the body looks for a storage place to put these toxins, where they can't do too much damage. The ideal storage place is fat tissue, because it does not play much of a role in the day-to-day functioning of the body. Accumulated toxins can be stored there safely without any risk of damage to vital organs such as the heart and the brain.

When someone goes on a calorie-restricted diet and starts to burn off fat tissue, the toxins that have been stored in these cells are released into the bloodstream. If the elimination system is functioning well, these toxins will be speedily and efficiently removed from the blood and body. However, if the elimination channels are not performing at their best, the increased toxic load can cause problems. Do you recall a time when you were on a diet and ended up feeling mentally sluggish, irritable or fatigued? One reason for experiencing uncomfortable side effects like these when on a diet is the uncontrolled release of accumulated toxins into the bloodstream and the inability of elimination channels to remove them quickly.

The blood is kept within a very tight alkaline range. The toxins that are released from fat cells are acidic. As these reach the bloodstream they create an overly acidic environment which needs to be rectified urgently. It is our system becomes acidic in this way that we experience all of the common dieting side effects such as grogginess or fatigue.

Avoiding Unpleasant Side Effects

There is a great deal that we can do to avoid having to experience these unsavoury side effects while we are losing weight. Given that a certain amount of acidic waste will inevitably be released, it will be helpful to take steps to keep the body alkaline. The foods that we choose to eat can have a very big impact in this respect. Wheat, high-protein foods and certain other grains leave an acidic residue when they are metabolized. Therefore these foods will increase the acidity of the body. On the other hand, all fruit and vegetables leave an alkaline residue. By cutting down our intake of acid-forming foods and replacing these with alkaline-forming foods we help to maintain an alkaline balance in the body. This is just one of the many reasons why you are encouraged to eat lots of fruit and vegetables on this plan.

The other aspect of this strategy to keep feeling great while losing weight is to help the elimination channels to work as efficiently as possible. It is vital to avoid becoming dehydrated. Water is needed for each of the parts of the elimination process. When we are dehydrated, the limited fluid that is available is either stuck where it shouldn't be (fluid retention) or is reserved for the most important bodily functions. In terms of our immediate survival, keeping the brain working is more important than servicing the digestive system so insufficient fluid intake impacts negatively on the digestive system. Chronic dehydration is one cause of constipation. When we are unable to remove waste products through this route we both overburden the other parts of our elimination system and increase the likelihood of the body becoming overly acidic. There are several easy steps we can take to improve our elimination channels. These are outlined in Chapter Seven.

Some Comments on Calories

By now, I hope I've convinced you that weight loss isn't just about calorie counting. The process is more complex than that. To lose weight healthily and permanently we need to work with a combination of elements such as our metabolism and keeping our elimination channels clear. Of course, calories cannot be dismissed altogether. Consuming

10,000 calories a day, every day, even if it is all really healthy food, is going to stop you losing weight.

If you like to think in terms of calories, here are some ball park figures. The average woman uses up about 2,000 calories/8,360 kilojoules per day while the average man uses around 2,500 calories/10,450 kilojoules per day. Your personal requirements may be slightly less or slightly more, depending on your level of physical activity. When your diet consists of healthy foods a daily intake of roughly 1700 calories/7,106 kilojoules for women and 2200 calories/9,196 kilojoules for men can still produce weight loss. This means that you can have three good meals per day, plus a couple of healthy snacks. But, as was discussed earlier, not all calories are the same. It is the type of food that you eat rather than the precise number of calories that can make the big difference between success or failure. You don't need to count calories on this plan. If you follow the meal plans you will getting approximately this level of calorie intake. So feel free to throw those calorie charts away and shift to a healthier way of eating, which will allow you to lose weight without skipping meals or feeling deprived.

chapter 3

Wheat – Your Weight and Your Health

Before reading on, I'd like you to conduct a little experiment. Grab a pen and a piece of paper and write down everything that you've eaten over the past two days. Include the main meals plus all the snacks. Now have a look at this list and beside each item write down the principal ingredients it contains. Don't worry, you don't have to be a food scientist to do this. There is no need to make a note of every single ingredient in a precise fashion; just record the main ingredients of each meal and snack. For example, if last night's evening meal was pasta with clams in a cream sauce, then the principal ingredients would be wheat (pasta), seafood and dairy (milk, cream).

Analysing the foods that you eat in this way can be extremely interesting. The list that you have just made can give you some important information regarding the main food groups that you normally consume (unless, of course, your eating habits on the last two days have been totally different from your usual pattern, in which case start again with more typical meals). It's also worthwhile to break down the ingredients of any favourite meals that you eat regularly but which are not already on your list.

How Much Wheat Do We Eat?

A typical food diary for the majority of people living in Europe and North America will usually consist of just three or four primary ingredients which show up again and again. One of these main ingredients is wheat. When I have asked clients to think about their food in this way they are usually genuinely surprised to discover how frequently they are eating this food. This is because wheat is packaged and processed into so many different food products that we may not realise that what we had for breakfast and what we had for dinner is essentially the same thing, just flavoured differently! As there is not much to do while waiting in line at the supermarket (and because I suffer from a very low boredom threshold), I often pass the time by looking at the contents of fellow shoppers' trolleys. I do just what I've suggested you try, and think about what each product is made from. I scan the items and, even though they may look like completely different foods, I inevitably find that a great many of our regular food purchases contain high levels of wheat. The next time you are in the supermarket, take a stroll along the aisle that contains the breakfast cereals. It might seem impressive that we have such an amazing range to choose from. However, the majority of cereals contain only one main ingredient. No prizes for guessing what that ingredient is!

This doesn't just apply to breakfast cereals. The predominance of wheat is found in several sections of the supermarket. For example, British shoppers have the choice of around two hundred varieties of bread made from wheat flour, plus all the different types of rolls, buns, croissants, baps and muffins. Every day, ten million loaves of bread are sold which suggests that on average each person consumes about four slices of bread per day.

A typical shopping list includes many wheat-based items such as bread, crackers, crispbread, pancakes, pizza, pasta, doughnuts, pretzels, biscuits (cookies) and cakes. A typical day's menu for many people consists of wheat-based cereal or toast for breakfast, a sandwich at lunchtime, pasta or pizza for dinner and cookies, crackers and pretzels as snacks. Further, many processed foods such as canned soups and sauces contain added wheat.

The Value of Variety

One of the core principles of creating a diet designed to support our health and well-being is that it should consist of a variety of different foods. The benefit of this is simple: the more varied the diet, the more likely we are to get the whole spectrum of nutrients that our body needs. Given that so many foods contain the same ingredients, it is actually quite difficult to achieve this. The next time you are waiting in line at the supermarket take a sneaky look at what others are buying. Break the whole shopping basket down into proportions for each food group. What percentage consists of fruit and vegetables? How much consists of meat and fish? How many products have chemicals added to them? How many products contain wheat, dairy foods (milk, cheese) or refined sugar? Unless the area where you live is very different to mine you will probably find that at least half of the items in most people's shopping trolleys contain wheat, dairy products, sugar and chemicals.

I don't believe that people actively go out of their way to purchase such foods. The problem is that we don't have as much choice as we think. A supermarket might stock two thousand food products, but when these are broken down into their basic elements, we find the same ingredients cropping up again and again. We, the consumers, are not to blame for this state of affairs. It is the food manufacturers, who appear to have a desire to stick to using the same ingredients in all types of foods, that might benefit from reflecting upon how this situation affects the nation's health.

Not as Healthy as We Think

What is wrong with eating wheat at every meal? Isn't it supposed to be a healthy food? Wheat has the image of being nutritious and wholesome. Healthy eating guidelines produced by government bodies in both Britain and America urge us to eat several portions of wheat-based foods such as bread and pasta each day. Wheat is considered to be good for us because it supplies carbohydrates and is supposedly a good source of dietary fibre.

We definitely need carbohydrates in our diet, they are the body's favourite source of energy. But, as I have already stated, not all carbohydrates are the same. Some are very good at supporting our health and well-being. Others disrupt the metabolism. Just because a food is high in carbohydrates doesn't automatically mean that it is good for us. Many carbohydrate foods contain very little that is of nutritional value. Unfortunately a lot of foods that contain wheat fall into this category.

Fibre is also an extremely important part of a healthy diet. But again, not all fibre is the same. Dietary fibre comes in several different forms and is found in a wide variety of foods. For many people, wheat fibre is not the best choice.

The Staff of Life

Wheat has the image of being a traditional food. We might think of our grandmothers kneading dough and baking bread or reflect on the phrase 'the staff of life'. Wheat has been part of the diet of Europeans and North Americans for several hundred years, but it is only relatively recently that we have started to consume this grain in such vast quantities. Since the arrival of both mass food production and supermarkets about fifty years ago the amount of wheat in an average diet has increased considerably. In the USA pasta, cereals, bagels, pretzels and pizza have been among the fastest growing food products during the last decade.

However, the wheat that we eat nowadays bears little resemblance to the grain our grandmothers would have used for baking. The amount of synthetic chemicals used by farmers has increased tremendously during the past seventy-five years. So even before wheat has been taken from the fields it has been exposed to high levels of insecticides, fungicides and similar chemicals. Modern wheat undergoes a bewildering array of processes before it is used in the products we purchase. The germ, which is a part of the wheat grain that is actually quite good for us as it is high in vitamin E and many of the B vitamins, is removed because it turns rancid very quickly and would therefore spoil the flour.

Bran, the fibre part of the grain, is also removed during most milling processes as the majority of the wheat products we consume are made with white flour.

The Chemical Cocktail

Until about fifty years ago wheat flour, like wine, would be stored for months in a warehouse to allow it to age. This ageing period improved the flavour. Nowadays, to save storage costs and time, manufacturers have developed chemical oxidizing agents such as potassium bromate which are added to the flour to age the wheat within 48 hours. Then the naturally occurring yellow pigmentation of the flour is bleached with chemicals such as benzoyl peroxide to turn it white, as this is considered more appealing. The bleaching agent needs to be neutralized by the addition of yet another chemical (such as calcium carbonate, which is chalk). It is also common practice to irradiate wheat in order to avoid contamination by insects. Finally, preservatives and conditioners are added to the flour to help improve the texture.

All the chemicals used in the flour-making process are, to use the terminology of the American Food and Drug Administration, 'generally regarded as safe', but it is nevertheless the case that by the time a product containing wheat reaches the supermarket shelves, the grain is in a very different form to how it started out. Most of the vitamins and minerals that were originally present have been lost during the milling and production process. In an attempt to compensate for this, manufacturers add synthetic vitamins and minerals to the flour. The problem with this strategy is that the nutrients added are produced from artificial ingredients, which the body has great difficulty assimilating, so many of the added nutrients are simply not absorbed. The amount of nutrition that we get from many wheat-based foods, including cereals and pasta, is often rather poor.

If we are keen to support our overall health and well-being, a diet containing high levels of wheat-based products is not the answer. Refined carbohydrates, which include many wheat-based products, will not support our weight-loss efforts. Furthermore, eating this same grain at every meal, as many people do, can be a factor in developing an intolerance to wheat.

The Fibre Debate

Fibre is good for us. It improves the functioning of the colon, which means that there is less likelihood of constipation or similar digestive disorders. A higher intake of fibre is also associated with a lower level of blood lipids, which reduces the risk of heart disease. Fibre can also protect against colon, breast and prostate cancer. Finally, several scientific studies have shown a link between fibre intake and weight. The greater level of fibre in the diet, the easier it can be to shed excess pounds.

Most products containing wheat contribute very little fibre as they are made from white flour, which has had the bran removed. For example, 100g of white bread yields only 2.3g of fibre. From this, we might assume that wholemeal or wholewheat products, which haven't had the fibre removed, must be better for us. This is not necessarily so. Many individuals turn to cereals such as wheat bran in an attempt to improve their digestive systems. Wheat bran contains 32.3g of fibre per 100g. As fibre is associated with digestive function, it would seem unlikely that anyone eating a food with those levels would be bothered by constipation, but for a great many people wheat bran actually increases constipation and also causes digestive discomfort such as abdominal bloating and flatulence. Once the wheat bran is removed and alternative sources of fibre are substituted for it, digestive health becomes much improved.

Forms of Fibre

Fibre can be soluble or insoluble. Each form has a different effect on the digestive system. All grains contain a mixture of both insoluble and soluble fibre. Wheat bran, however, contains a very high percentage of insoluble fibre. Many people choose white bread instead of wholemeal (wholewheat) because they find the latter is much more difficult to digest and causes bloating and abdominal discomfort. It seems that the insoluble fibre found in wheat bran is very abrasive to the colon. The same irritation does not occur with other whole grains that contain lower amounts of insoluble fibre.

Phytates are also found in the fibre of grains. These are chemical substances that bind with minerals such as calcium, iron, zinc and copper.

Wheat contains a high level of phytates relative to many other grains. A bowl of wheat bran with milk in the morning will not provide us with much calcium because the mineral cannot be absorbed. Instead, the calcium binds with the phytates and is eliminated through the digestive tract. Consuming a diet high in phytates can lead to deficiencies of these key nutrients.

There are plenty of alternative foods we can turn to in order to get our daily supply of dietary fibre without having to endure the problems associated with insoluble fibre or phytates. Most other grains provide us with a greater percentage of soluble fibre, which is much kinder to the digestive tract. Oats and oat bran are much better than wheat bran for breakfast. Oat bran contains 15.4g of fibre per 100g but as most of this is soluble, the body can process it much more easily. Other foods that are excellent sources of soluble fibre are broad (lima) beans, kidney beans, soya beans, lentils and chickpeas. Fruit and vegetables rank highly as well. All of these foods are nutritious. They are all also excellent foods to eat on a weight loss plan. As you will see in the coming chapters, these foods are helpful in many ways, including providing support to help avoid cravings.

Food Allergy versus Food Intolerance

Food intolerance and food allergy are not the same thing. A food allergy produces an immediate and extreme physical reaction as soon as the allergic person comes into contact with the offending food. Shellfish and peanuts are common culprits. The food doesn't even need to be swallowed; sometimes just having it come into contact with the tongue or lips can produce a reaction. Allergy can produce a host of dangerous symptoms such as swelling of the throat and anaphylactic shock. When we have a food allergy it remains with us forever. We need to scrupulously avoid that particular food for life.

Food intolerance is a different type of condition. When an allergy is triggered the response is immediate and the symptoms are potentially life-threatening. Food intolerance, on the other hand, is associated with milder symptoms that generally take longer to manifest themselves. These may not necessarily occur as soon as the culprit food is eaten; it can take up to two days for the symptoms to emerge. This time-lag between eating the offending food and experiencing the effect makes the link between the two very difficult to spot. Also, because the cluster of symptoms that somebody may be experiencing can be so varied there may be no clear connection with a specific food. To further complicate matters, different symptoms can also appear at different times in a seemingly random pattern. Food intolerance can be difficult to diagnose. The symptoms can persist for a long time without a connection to the offending food being made.

Some Symptoms of Food Intolerance

A host of symptoms and medical conditions have been associated with intolerance. These include migraines, rheumatoid arthritis, asthma and even psychological conditions such as depression. Irritable bowel syndrome (IBS), which affects one in four people in Britain, has been found to be strongly linked to food intolerance, in particular to wheat or dairy products. Symptoms of IBS include constipation, diarrhoea, abdominal pain and bloating. Several research studies conducted at Addenbrooke's Hospital in Cambridge, England have reported that in a large proportion of cases these symptoms clear up once the offending food, which is often wheat, is removed from the diet.

When food intolerance is present it can be much more difficult to lose weight. There are several reasons for this. A somewhat paradoxical aspect of food intolerance is that we often crave the culprit food. Dr Jonathan Brostoff, who has done some pioneering work in this area, estimates that 50 per cent of people with food intolerance crave the food or foods to which they are intolerant. 'Withdrawal symptoms' often kick in if the food is not eaten regularly. This type of craving can significantly hamper our weight loss efforts even if we are absolutely determined to stick to a diet. For some people this form of craving can be extremely powerful, resulting in periods of binge eating.

Food intolerance is also associated with excess fluid retention which will not shift even when we are reducing our calorie intake. Chapter Five looks at both these problems in more depth.

Because it is difficult to recognize food intolerance, the extent of this problem throughout the population is very difficult to assess scientifically. However, the limited number of studies that have been done in this field suggest that the overall number of people who are experiencing food intolerance is on the increase.

Causes of Food Intolerance

There are no conclusive scientific explanations as to the causes of food intolerance, because the biochemical mechanisms involved are not totally understood. However, two combined factors seem to be strongly implicated. The first suggests that simply eating a particular food too often can be a trigger. Most of the medical specialists who work in this field agree that eating the same food over and over again is a major contributory factor in developing intolerance. As wheat is such a regular part of the typical diet it is not surprising that this food is often a culprit.

It is not clear why frequently eating the same food can provoke intolerance, but a current widely held theory is that this over-consumption causes the body's digestive enzymes to malfunction. The food is not digested properly and this provokes health problems. The structure of the food concerned is therefore important. Foods which are digested easily (such as fruit) can be eaten frequently without provoking a disturbance in the digestive enzymes. Foods which are more difficult to digest, including wheat, are likely to cause an intolerance if eaten too often. As the wheat grain that we eat today is very different from the grain that was eaten by our ancestors, it may also be the case that the specific structure of the current grain is very difficult for the body's enzymes to process effectively.

The digestive system is also involved in food intolerance in another way. The nutrients we derive from food are absorbed into the body from the small intestine. Molecules are transported through the wall of the small intestine and subsequently used by the body. The large intestine (colon) does not play much of a role in the absorption process, so the walls of the colon are much stronger ensuring, that very little is absorbed back into the body.

Leaky Gut

If the digestive system is not in perfect health the colon wall may become more permeable. This increased permeability (often called 'leaky gut') allows food molecules to seep through the colon wall into the blood and bodily fluids. As these broken-down food molecules are not supposed to get into these areas the immune system perceives them as invaders and triggers a host of reactions to eliminate them. It is this immune response that precipitates the symptoms that arise with intolerance. Dr Brostoff suggests that increased chemical exposure (both from food additives and pollutants in the environment) and frequent use of antibiotics (which disturb the delicate bacteria living in the gut) are principal factors that can increase gut permeability and therefore make an individual susceptible to food intolerance.

The link between food intolerance and digestive function is very important and is good news in that it suggests that a food intolerance, unlike an allergy, does not have to be for life. By avoiding the culprit food for a period of time and simultaneously taking steps to improve the health of the digestive system we should find that in the longer-term we can tolerate small amounts of the offending food without difficulty. Nobody should suffer from food intolerance for years and years. When the correct steps are taken to address the problem, the majority of people find that it resolves itself quite quickly. The ability to lose weight is also linked with the health of the digestive system. For both of these reasons, Chapter Six is devoted to outlining steps that can be taken to improve digestive health.

Specific Problem Areas

Two components of the wheat grain are linked with an intolerance to this food. The bran can irritate the digestive tract (especially the colon), causing symptoms such as bloating, constipation and/or diarrhoea. Many people find that these symptoms are not so severe when they eat foods based on white (rather than wholemeal (wholewheat)) flour, as the bran content is significantly reduced or negligible. The protein portion of wheat is also implicated in an intolerance problem. Wheat protein (gluten) is made up of gliadin and glutenin. Gliadin, which is not easily digested, is particularly associated with intolerance symptoms. Digestive enzymes are important for the breakdown of protein molecules, but frequent consumption of the same food can cause these enzymes to function poorly. When the colon has become permeable, these protein molecules can seep through into the body and trigger an immune system response. Gliadin is present in all types of flour so switching to white flour won't improve the situation.

Gluten is also present in the other grains, namely oats, barley and rye, but the chemical structure of the protein molecules is different in each. Furthermore, there is significantly less gluten in the other three grains than there is in wheat. Many people who are intolerant to wheat find that they can still eat oats, barley and rye without experiencing any adverse side effects. Some people however, are sensitive to the gluten from whichever source, even if coeliac disease is not present.

Coeliac Disease

Wheat intolerance is not to be confused with coeliac disease. Coeliac disease is a condition where gluten/gliadin irritates the lining of the colon wall severely causing pain and symptoms such as diarrhoea. The condition generally lasts for life and all gluten-containing grains must be scrupulously avoided.

In addition to those who are diagnosed with coeliac disease, there seems to be a sub-set of people who test negative for the disorder but who nonetheless find that their digestive problems improve – or even disappear – when they eliminate from their diet grains that contain gluten. If your symptoms include frequent diarrhoea and intestinal discomfort and there is no improvement when wheat is removed from your diet, you could experiment to see whether avoiding the other sources of gluten (oats, barley and rye) makes a difference. However, it is essential that you also see your doctor, so that the cause of this problem can be properly investigated.

Testing for Wheat Intolerance

There are a number of biochemical tests that can indicate if an intolerance is present. Most of these are quite expensive and the accuracy of some approaches is doubtful. Ultimately, the most effective (and cheapest) way of determining an intolerance is to remove the suspect food from your diet for a period of four weeks and monitor the results. In assessing an intolerance, it can also be useful to look at symptoms. The questionnaire below will help you do just that. It contains a list of symptoms that have been found to be associated with wheat intolerance. Please note however, that some of these symptoms could indicate a medical problem, so it is recommended that you also see your doctor. It is not a good idea to allow any physical symptom to persist without seeking the advice of a medically qualified professional.

If you answered 'yes' to seven or more of these questions then it is probable that you are intolerant to wheat. If you answered 'yes' at least four times then, even though you may not technically be intolerant, you could still benefit from eliminating wheat from your diet for a while. Intolerance, however, is a tricky thing to identify without com-

---

SELF TEST WHEAT INTOLERANCE QUESTIONNAIRE

1 My stomach feels bloated for no apparent reason **yes/no**
2 I get flatulence (gas) or indigestion quite regularly **yes/no**
3 I do *not* have a bowel movement at least once a day **yes/no**
4 I experience diarrhoea at least a few times every month **yes/no**
5 I get fluid retention, especially before a period **yes/no**
6 I feel really groggy when I wake up in the morning **yes/no**
7 I often feel really tired even though I get enough sleep **yes/no**
8 I experience 'brain fog' or find it difficult to concentrate **yes/no**
9 I experience headaches or migraines **yes/no**
10 My joints and/or my muscles ache **yes/no**
11 I have eczema, acne or a similar skin condition **yes/no**
12 I find that I crave wheat-containing foods **yes/no**
13 My energy can slump after eating pasta, bread, or pizza **yes/no**
14 My weight can fluctuate up and down for no obvious reason **yes/no**
15 I get energy dips at various points of the day **yes/no**

prehensive biochemical tests. It's a bit like being a detective – weighing up all the clues and then arriving at an educated and experienced conclusion as to who or what is the most likely suspect. Different clues generally combine to create a pattern, or a specific collection of symptoms, which individually might not mean much but together can be highly significant.

To help you to make a more detailed assessment of whether you may have a problem with wheat I would usually expect you to have answered 'yes' to at least one of the first five questions or at least one of the final four questions (12 to 15). If this is not the case, affirmative answers to the other symptoms listed in the middle section (6 to 11) such as brain fog or feeling really tired may not be related to wheat intolerance at all. But when positive responses to questions 6 to 11 are combined with positive responses from either the first and/or the last part of the questionnaire, the evidence would seem to indicate quite strongly that your system may have difficulty in handling wheat.

Wheat and Your Weight

A few years before I trained as a nutritionist I spent three weeks in China. During that period I naturally lost 4kg/7lb and the stomach bloating that I often experienced totally disappeared. On top of that I felt absolutely fantastic and had loads of energy. My time in China was with an organized tour, so there was no shortage of food. We were provided with three large meals per day, plus snacks and fruit that we bought ourselves. I wasn't trying to lose weight so I was eating generous portions at every meal. I had a similar experience a year later, when my partner and I visited Thailand. We both love Thai food so we did not restrict our food intake in any way. Again I lost weight, felt great and had no stomach bloating. It was only later, during my training, that I made the connection between what I'd been eating on these trips and the change in my well-being. I had naturally been following a wheat-free diet, because this is the norm for people in these regions. Chinese and South-East Asian food also contains a lot less fat than Western fare but, as I have never been a lover of fatty food, I doubt that this was a factor in my weight loss.

As you have seen in this chapter, there are several reasons why foods that contain wheat are not ideal on a weight-loss plan. And for some people, discovering that they have a wheat intolerance can be the key to finally losing those extra pounds.

Keith, a stockbroker friend of mine who was about 8.2kg/18lbs overweight, lost an amazing 4.5kg/10lb within a week of removing wheat from his diet. Of course, most of this drop in weight was due to the elimination of excess fluid. However, he felt so inspired and energized by this experience that it motivated him to continue his weight-loss plan until he reached his ideal weight. He also felt motivated to start exercising again, so within about two months he had achieved a much higher level of fitness and vitality. While removing an offending food can bring excellent results, it is still very important to take steps to strengthen the body, so that the intolerance problem is sorted out and that situation does not recur in the future.

chapter 4

Say Goodbye
to Cravings

Have you reached the point where you are convinced that you must simply have been born with a lousy willpower when it comes to food? Do you start the day enthusiastic and strongly committed to your weight-loss goals only to be overcome with an irresistible urge to reach for a bar of chocolate by mid-afternoon? Well, you may be giving yourself a hard time for nothing. Cravings such as these are not always 'all in the mind' or simply indicative of a weak willpower. Instead, they are often purely physical in nature. This is good news because if cravings are the result of physical mechanisms, there must be ways that we can work effectively with these processes. We don't need to have an iron will to achieve successful weight loss, and we can stop feeling guilty and worthless because we have succumbed to cravings in the past.

This chapter looks at the most common reason for food cravings and includes some straightforward guidelines that will help you to overcome this problem once and for all. It introduces another of the star players of your weight-loss team; a strategy that will provide tremendous support to your metabolic process and increase the rate at which you burn off fat.

There are a few other nutritional triggers that can also lead to food cravings. These are discussed in depth in the following chapter.

Blood Sugar Balance

The most likely reason for experiencing cravings or succumbing to overeating is a blood sugar imbalance. This is not a medical condition, like diabetes; it is an indicator that while this system is functioning it is not functioning as well as it should. As blood sugar problems are extremely common, I have provided you with a set of questions designed to help you assess whether or not this might apply to you. Take a couple of minutes to go through these questions, before reading any further, but please remember that the self-tests in this book are only designed as helpful indicators of nutritional conditions and should never be regarded as a substitute for proper medical advice.

Juliet's story is a very good example of how a blood sugar problem can hamper any attempt at weight loss and simultaneously make life a bit of a

BLOOD SUGAR BALANCE ASSESSMENT

1 I experience an energy drop late morning and/or mid-afternoon
yes/no
2 I feel dizzy and nauseous if I go for a few hours without food
yes/no
3 I sometimes find myself feeling panicky for no reason **yes/no**
4 I often feel light-headed and 'spaced out' **yes/no**
5 I can get irritable or aggressive if I haven't eaten for a while
yes/no
6 Sometimes I feel so ravenous that I grab the first thing available
yes/no
7 Without warning I can feel depressed or on the verge of tears
yes/no
8 I don't have enough energy to exercise regularly **yes/no**
9 The foods I most crave are carbohydrates (e.g., sugar, bread)
yes/no
10 I consume coffee to give myself a lift when my energy is low
yes/no
11 I sometimes lose concentration or find it hard to think clearly
yes/no
12 Many of these symptoms get worse just before my period **yes/no**

misery. Juliet, a 34-year-old self-employed graphic designer, complained of a lack of energy, frequent emotional fluctuations, premenstrual problems and headaches. Every afternoon she would feel so tired and drained that she needed to stop work to have a two-hour sleep. She was counting calories and going to the gym three times a week but the 19kg/42lb she had gained in the past five years stubbornly refused to budge.

A typical day's menu for Juliet consisted of cornflakes for breakfast, a ham sandwich for lunch (made with white bread) and fish cakes with chips or French fries for dinner. During the run-up to her period she had a strong craving for carbohydrates such as bread, biscuits or cookies and sweets (candy).

After making some dietary changes designed to support her blood sugar balance and correct a range of nutritional deficiencies, Juliet noticed that her health improved considerably. Her symptoms cleared up and the excess pounds started to drop off steadily. Within a few weeks she had a great deal more energy. She no longer needed to sleep in the afternoon and the headaches and emotional ups-and-downs disappeared. The premenstrual cravings cleared up virtually immediately and the other premenstrual problems were gone after a couple of months. Juliet's new eating plan gave her more calories each day than she had been eating before, but the increase actively helped her lose weight. This was because the foods she was now eating provided calories in a form that helped her body to burn fat and *improved* the functioning of her metabolic system. Juliet eventually reached her ideal weight and managed to maintain this weight in the long-term.

If you have answered 'yes' to at least five of the questions on the self-test assessment, your blood sugar balance could probably do with some support. You certainly won't be alone in this; any nutritionist would tell you that blood sugar problems are one of the most frequent conditions that they see. This is because many of the foods that we eat regularly do an incredibly bad job supporting our blood sugar. Modern lifestyles, which are characterized by high levels of stress and long working hours, also put added strain on the delicate mechanism that regulates blood sugar. Fortunately, you don't need to make a massive adjustment to your eating patterns to improve your blood sugar balance. Simple changes can produce noticeable improvements very quickly, usually within a couple of weeks. These changes will also help your metabolism to work efficiently, thereby making weight loss easier.

How the System Works

Blood sugar consists of glucose, which constantly circulates through the body to provide muscles and organs with the energy they need for their daily activities. Carbohydrates are the body's favourite source of energy, as they can be converted into glucose very efficiently. Fats are quite a good source of fuel, ranking second to carbohydrates, but protein foods cannot be converted into energy very easily; instead their main purpose is to rebuild and repair the body.

A stable blood sugar – which will help us to avoid cravings, shed extra pounds easily and give us high levels of energy – can only be created by having the optimum balance of carbohydrates, fats and proteins in our diet. Not all types of carbohydrates will support us in this goal. Some carbohydrates are extremely good at balancing blood sugar. Others can actually provoke a blood sugar problem. Given the foods that are available on supermarket shelves, it isn't surprising that many of us fail to get the balance right. Instead, we often end up with a diet that consists of lots of the wrong type of carbohydrates, rather too much protein, too much of the wrong type of fat and virtually none of the essential healthy fats. Stress, drinking lots of coffee and habits such as regularly skipping meals also come into the equation. With these combined factors we create the ideal conditions for a blood sugar problem to develop.

The Balancing Act

Blood sugar is in perfect balance when we are able to keep the blood's glucose levels stable within an optimum range throughout the day. When this happens, the body, emotions and mind can perform at their best. The metabolism is supported and efforts at weight loss are likely to be successful. We are less likely to experience cravings or want to overeat. When blood sugar is imbalanced – either too high or too low – we experience problems. When it is too high, we can feel 'wired' or stressed and when it is too low we are at that dangerous point where we can become overcome with cravings and the desire to binge.

A robust and healthy blood sugar mechanism can cope with the occasional bar of chocolate without experiencing any ill-effects. Although our blood glucose will rapidly rise beyond the optimum range after eating the confectionery (due to the speed at which the refined sugar has been converted by the body), the system will be able to bring it back to a healthy range within a short time. But when the blood sugar mechanism is not working well the act of eating the chocolate (especially on an empty stomach) can throw the whole system into chaos.

Eating a diet high in refined carbohydrates, skipping meals, experiencing stress or drinking lots of coffee can result in the blood sugar mechanism becoming 'trigger happy'. Frequently going on calorie-counting diets can also provoke this type of reaction. The mechanisms involved in balancing blood sugar levels are unable to hold them steady, so they yo-yo up and down throughout the day. Whenever something like a biscuit or cookie is eaten the subsequent rise in blood sugar is interpreted as a serious threat by the blood sugar balancing mechanism. The mechanism overacts, and compensates by drawing too much glucose from the bloodstream, with the result that, after forty-five minutes or so, the blood sugar has fallen too low.

When Blood Sugar Plummets

When blood sugar has plummeted like this we generally start to feel pretty lousy. We may find ourselves unable to think clearly or may suddenly feel irritable or depressed. Low blood sugar is perceived by the body as a highly dangerous situation which needs to be rectified at once. It responds by releasing chemicals which urge us to eat anything, as long as it's immediately, so that our glucose levels can be restored to normal. It is at times like these, when our blood sugar has slumped too low, that cravings kick in with tremendous force.

When we are in this state all of our commitment to weight loss can fly out of the window because we are literally not thinking clearly. Indeed, because of the lack of glucose, brain function is well below par and concerned with only one thing; how to replenish the depleted glucose stores.

A research team at the University of Florida in the US have found that it takes ten minutes from the time you start eating for the brain to signal that it is full and thereby turn off the 'food urgently required' sign. If you are overweight, the time it takes for your brain to produce this signal can be even longer. Ten minutes is a long time to be gripped by strong cravings. It is possible, even without fully realising what we are doing, to consume a lot of food during this period.

Carbohydrate Cravings

To make matters worse, what we tend to crave when blood sugar levels have taken a dive are foods such as refined carbohydrates (biscuits, cookies, white bread, sugar) because these are the ones that will push our blood sugar up very quickly. Although eating these foods will make us feel better for a short while, the speed at which they are converted into glucose will result in the blood sugar shooting up again. This provokes two reactions. First, the balancing mechanism leaps into action to remove the excess glucose from the blood. This extra energy has to go somewhere, so as soon as the limited storage space in the liver is full, the body has no option but to convert it directly into fat. Second, because the balancing mechanism is trigger happy, too much glucose is removed from the blood, and within an hour or so, we are back where we started, with low blood sugar. The familiar no-energy state prompts us to eat again, and the cycle starts once more. This can happen several times during the day and is why we can alternate between feeling energetic one minute and absolutely exhausted the next.

When the blood sugar is unstable in this way, we are much more likely to gain weight on fewer calories or find it very hard to lose weight. This is because of the link between blood sugar and the two sets of appetite control hormones that were mentioned in Chapter Two. These create conditions that mean any time blood sugar goes above the optimum range (like after eating a bar of chocolate) the excess glucose is quickly converted into fat tissue.

It is not just high-sugar foods such as sweets (candy) that are a problem. Unfortunately, many of the foods we usually consider quite healthy can disrupt blood sugar balance as well. Basically, any food that is refined or highly processed will be converted by the body into glucose very quickly, thus pushing our blood sugar beyond the optimum range. Most breakfast cereals fall into this category. This has the effect of making us feel voraciously hungry by mid-morning and we may also become aware that we are not functioning at top speed. The energy in the breakfast cereal reached the bloodstream hours ago, so by 11am blood sugar has become seriously low and we reach for biscuits, cookies or potato crisps (chips) in a desperate attempt to feel human again.

Stress and Stimulants

Stress and stimulants can also play havoc with our blood sugar balance. Whenever we feel stressed (in the sense of having too many things to do, pushing ourselves without a break, frequently getting angry and frustrated or worrying excessively) we trigger a surge in our blood sugar. Stored glucose (glycogen) is released by the liver and muscles and delivered to the bloodstream so we have plenty of energy to deal with the stressful situation. As we seldom deal with modern-day stress with physical activity (unlike primitive man, who would fight or take flight) the high blood sugar remains where it is. This provokes exactly the same situation as when we eat a refined carbohydrate food; biochemical mechanisms are required to bring the glucose down to an acceptable level.

Frequent stress places great strain on mechanisms for maintaining stable blood sugar levels perpetuating a trigger-happy, unbalanced system. Ironically, when blood sugar is unstable, we become much less resilient at handling day-to-day pressures. When we are feeling exhausted or our emotions are fluctuating wildly it is easy to get problems out of perspective. This creates another vicious cycle: we get stressed, which perpetuates blood sugar problems, which means we get even more stressed, which strains our blood sugar yet again, and so on. By following a diet that supports our blood sugar we can break this cycle and take control of life again.

A useful method for determining whether a particular carbohydrate food supports or disrupts the blood sugar balance is found in the

THE CAFFEINE HIT

In terms of blood sugar levels, the body reacts to caffeine – in coffee, tea, chocolate and many cola drinks – just as it does to stress. The reason we feel perky for a short while after drinking a cup of coffee is mainly because blood sugar levels have increased. An hour or so later, however, we experience that familiar energy slump once more.

Glycemic Index, which provides a numerical value for each food listed, based on how quickly that food is converted into glucose. If the value is high, the food is converted into blood glucose very quickly and can cause havoc with blood sugar levels. This type of food is termed 'fast-releasing'. Conversely, foods with low scores are slow-releasing. They help to create stable blood sugar levels by drip feeding small amounts of glucose into the bloodstream over a period of time, so we always have plenty of energy and our blood sugar remains in the optimum range.

As a general rule, consider any food that is highly processed or that contains a lot of refined sugar to be fast-releasing and therefore disrup-

GLYCEMIC INDEX FOR COMMON FOODS

Fast Releasing

sucrose (white sugar)	doughnuts *	croissants *
lucozade	mashed or baked potato	fizzy drinks
Cornflakes	rice cakes	cream of wheat *
French fries	Rice Crispies	biscuits (cookies) *
wheat bread *	rice, white	puffed crispbread *
bagels *	dates	macaroni & cheese *
jams & marmalade	honey	pizza, cheese *
		confectionery*

Moderate releasing

porridge	bananas	potato, boiled
oat bran	raisins & sultanas	ice cream, low fat
wheat-free muesli	melon	oranges & orange juice
sweet potato	wheat Bran *	sweet corn
rice, brown	baked beans, canned	carrots

Slow releasing

soya beans	kidney beans	apples & apple juice
cherries	butter beans	rice bran
fructose (fruit sugar)	yogurt, low-fat	pearl barley
soya milk	chickpeas	dried apricots
lentils	rye flakes & rye bread	split peas

* Contains wheat.

tive to your sugar balance. These are foods that you should avoid as much as possible. As most of these foods are pretty much devoid of any nutritional value you won't be missing much. Also, get into the habit, when you are shopping, of reading the ingredients label on products. Many processed foods contain hidden sugar. Ingredients such as maltose, corn syrup or dextrose are all forms of fast-releasing sugars, so it is probably wise to leave products with these ingredients on the supermarket shelf.

Complex Carbohydrates

Foods that are close to their natural state when we eat them are usually slow-releasing, which means they will *improve* your blood sugar balance. Most complex carbohydrates fall into this category. Beans, lentils and chickpeas are prime examples and should be eaten frequently. It is important to note, however, that how the food is cooked can affect how quickly the energy will be released. For example, baked or mashed potatoes are fast-releasing while boiled potatoes are moderate. In all other respects, a baked potato is a healthy choice that is easy to prepare so the best thing to do is combine it with a slower-releasing food such as baked beans or hummus. If you eat the skin of the potato you can also make it more slow-releasing, due to the added fibre content.

You might imagine fruit to be fast-releasing food, as it is naturally sweet and is digested easily. However most fruit (except bananas, grapes and oranges which are moderate-releasing) are slow-releasing. The same applies to fruit juice such as apple or grapefruit, as long as you prepare it yourself. This does not necessarily hold true for commercially-prepared juices, which often contain added sugar.

Steps to Success

If most of the carbohydrates you eat come from the slow- and moderate-releasing categories (essentially all complex carbohydrate foods) your blood sugar balance will improve quickly. It is also worthwhile looking at the level of stimulants you consume. If you currently drink a lot of coffee, tea or cola, cut down slowly so that you avoid withdrawal symptoms such as headaches. Herbal teas make great alternatives to coffee without the disruptive effects.

Taking steps to manage stress levels is equally important. Although it might not be possible to get away from all life's pressures, it is possible to learn to deal with them effectively so that stress levels are reduced.

A further step you can take to improve your blood sugar balance is to eat slow-releasing carbohydrates with small amounts of protein. Vegetarian protein works best in this regard, as it does not put too much strain on the digestive system. For example, adding a few tablespoons of yogurt to your breakfast porridge makes a meal that will give you energy for the whole morning, eliminating the 11 o'clock urge to raid the biscuit (cookie) tin. Nuts and seeds, which naturally combine protein and slow-releasing carbohydrates, make ideal snacks for eating between meals. Not only do they do a fantastic job in balancing blood sugar levels, but they also provide us with a good source of healthy fats and specific nutrients to support the metabolism. Seeds are therefore a key food in this weight-loss eating plan.

Spotting the Signals

Eating regularly and often is the only way that you can avoid experiencing blood sugar slumps. Ideally, you need to have three meals a day plus one or two snacks. The key to making this work is to follow your body's signals, rather than following a routine without paying attention to whether your body needs food or not. Your body will let you know when it would like some food and when it is satisfied. Only by paying attention to these messages will you regulate your food intake to the optimum level that is right for you.

Blood sugar is at its lowest first thing in the morning. This is why breakfast is an extremely important meal. A slow-releasing breakfast such as wheat-free muesli provides important fuel for the day ahead and jump-starts the metabolism. If you have no time for breakfast or you are not hungry first thing, the solution is to eat something as soon as you get to work or after you've dropped the children at school. Keep some healthy wheat-free cereals at your place of work and take a tub of yogurt with you, so you can have a bowl-full before you get involved in the day's activities.

It is also very helpful to always have access to healthy snacks while you are at work or out on the road. You can carry these in your bag or leave them in the car. Make it a habit to have a small amount of healthy snacks (see Chapter Eleven for suggestions) between meals so that you avoid the risk of your blood sugar falling to extremely low levels. The is particularly relevant if you work irregular hours, as your blood sugar mechanism will be working doubly hard to deal with the constant variation in schedule and eating patterns.

Tuning in

Start tuning in the unique signals your body gives you. Take a moment to reflect upon how you usually feel at different points of the day. You may realise that most days you feel pretty groggy at say, 4pm, the point where you reach for the doughnuts. You can short-circuit this pattern by eating a healthy snack at 3pm or 3.30pm. Do you nibble while preparing your children's evening meal and then still eat a full meal with your partner a couple of hours later? In this case, it might be worth eating lunch slightly later in the day and then giving yourself 15 minutes to sit down and eat a bowl of fruit salad with yogurt before you pick up the children from school. If you are not hungry, you will be much less likely to dip into the children's food.

Pay attention whenever you are feeling peckish (a physical sensation). This is the time to reach for a piece of fruit or a small handful of nuts and seeds. The only time you should not have the snack is if you are going to eat a full meal in the next 20 minutes. This might seem like a complete reversal of the eating pattern you might expect to adopt on a weight-loss programme, but if you continue past the peckish point by much more than twenty minutes you will end up in a full-blown low blood sugar situation. This just confuses your metabolism. It also makes it more likely that you will eat too much when you eventually do have a meal, and that the calories that you do consume are much more likely to be converted into fat. Having a small sensible snack before a meal helps you to avoid overeating when you do sit down to eat properly. And, as you will see in Chapter Five, there are specific foods that can do this job particularly well.

Feeling Pleasantly Peckish

This plan encourages you to become closely acquainted with your 'pleasantly peckish' feeling and use that as your signal to eat. Never let yourself get to the point of feeling ravenous, as this is highly counter-productive. Instead of following a routine when it comes to eating, trust and follow your body's signals. They will rarely be wrong.

Note that 'feeling peckish' refers to a genuine physical sensation, not the emotional feeling we get when we just fancy a bit of comfort food. Make this a guideline that you will follow on a daily basis: eat when you genuinely have a physical desire for food, but do not eat at all other times. The only time you should eat whether you are peckish or not is at breakfast (because your blood sugar will be low) or if you know for certain that you will not have access to food for the next few hours.

For example, you are normally hungry at 1pm, so you stop what you are doing to have lunch at this time. Today, you have an appointment at 12.30 which may last for an hour or two. In this instance it is best to eat lunch at 12 noon. You may not be very hungry, but it is better to have your meal at this time rather than waiting until the middle of the afternoon, by which point your blood sugar will have slumped. It's impossible to plan ahead for every eventuality, but you can take steps to manage your day to avoid fluctuations in your blood sugar and energy levels.

That Time of the Month

Many women find that they can be pretty disciplined with their diet most of the time except during the week before a period. At this time they are often overwhelmed with cravings for sweet foods and carbohydrates such as bread. Premenstrual symptoms may also include bloating, headaches, and psychological factors such as feeling depressed or irritable. When women are in the grip of hormones and feeling down it is very easy to fall into the trap of thinking that trying to lose weight is a waste of time.

The really good news is that following a diet designed to balance blood sugar usually has an extremely positive effect on premenstrual symptoms. If you do suffer from this problem, you can expect to notice a big improvement within a month or two. Removing a food to which you are intolerant from your diet can also make a difference to premenstrual problems. A third benefit of this eating plan is that the specific foods that you are encouraged to eat are ones that will also supply your body with the key nutrients that are important in balancing the menstrual cycle. These include the nuts and seeds which are high in the hormone-supporting nutrients magnesium, zinc, and essential fats.

No Need to Suffer

Premenstrual symptoms like the ones described earlier are not something that we have to endure. These can be addressed by making dietary and lifestyle changes. However, it is a natural consequence of the female hormonal cycle that women feel more introspective just before, and during, menstruation. This is quite natural and healthy. It reflects the cycles that happen throughout nature, such as the changing seasons and the ebb and flow of the tides. This time of the month is an opportunity to be more reflective especially as regards our emotional life. We may feel less sociable and need more private, peaceful time.

As we slow down and reflect upon our lives we become more aware of what is going on in our emotional world, and areas of dissatisfaction may surface. At other times of the month we won't be as aware of these aspects because the hormonal balance is making us more outward-focussed.

Maggie became depressed for a *week* every month, as regular as clockwork. This was because she would suddenly become excruciatingly aware of the aspects of her relationship that were not working well. After her period she would brighten up and say 'well, things are not that bad really' and continue as before. Whenever she went through the down phase, she would use comfort eating to try to alleviate the unpleasant feelings. Usually, however, this strategy only served to make Maggie feel worse, because eating lots of sweet foods made her feel physically bad and she felt frustrated with herself for not sticking to her weight-loss objectives. And, of course, eating these foods didn't make the uncomfortable feelings she was having about her relationship go away.

This cycle continued for several months until Maggie decided to pay attention to these internal messages. She left the children with her parents for a couple of weeks and went on holiday with her partner. They spent a lot of time discussing their relationship and worked out ways to bring back the sparkle and romance. Since their holiday the relationship has improved considerably and Maggie no longer feels depressed every month.

Listen to Your Feelings

Within Western culture we are urged to be happy· all the time. This image is portrayed in the movies, advertisements and magazines. Think of the adverts for washing powder. There's Mum, overjoyed at how amazingly white her whites have turned out! With images like these, it isn't surprising that some of us develop unrealistic expectations. However, if we are feeling down because of a specific situation, there is little value in ignoring these feelings or trying to make them go away by turning to chocolate. Negative feelings actually have a very valuable role to play.

If you put your finger in a candle flame, the sensation of pain would make you draw it away. Without the pain you might be seriously burned. So in this instance, pain is good. In the same way, feeling down or slightly depressed can be an important and healthy signal, telling us that we need to make some changes to our life. The reflective time to which women are naturally predisposed at the time of a period can be useful. We can embrace our natural rhythms by giving ourselves sufficient private time at this time of the month. It can be a great time to nurture ourselves in healthy ways, such as by spending an evening trying out new beauty treatments at home or curling up with a good book.

One way of working with any feelings or thoughts that surface during this time is to write them down. The process can help to bring clarity to our feelings and create new insights regarding changes we might make. The act of writing actually creates physical changes in the body. It releases some stress hormones and has a positive impact on our immune system. By expressing our feelings in this way we can short-circuit the desire to reach for the sweet foods, which would just make us feel worse in the long-run.

Comfort Eating

Of course, the desire to reach for sweet foods because we are feeling depressed can happen at any time of the month. I've never met anyone who hasn't turned to food at least once in their life when they were feeling low. It's a natural habit, as we associate food with nurturing and feeling good. However, if we continually follow this pattern we will never achieve the weight loss we desire.

Everyone has a different repertoire of strategies that they use to cope with difficult times and uncomfortable emotions. Some people turn to food. Over time, continually using the same strategy will turn it into a habit. However, habits can be changed easily once you recognize the behaviour and devise alternative strategies. If you are aware that you have a tendency to turn to food when you are feeling a bit low, all you need to do is take steps to break the pattern.

Alan, a hairdresser, came to see me because he wanted to lose weight. He confessed that he knew exactly what he needed to do, but said he just wanted to hear it from someone else. (This is a role I often find myself in!) Alan's main difficulty with weight loss was that he would overeat whenever he felt down or stressed. I recommended two strategies for him to follow. He needed to adopt a blood sugar balancing diet so that the physical cravings for food were reduced. He also needed to develop different ways of dealing with his emotional needs. Instead of reaching for the cookies every time he felt depressed I suggested he ask his wife for a hug, spend five minutes away from clients to do a relaxation exercise or write down his feelings in a journal.

Over a period of a few weeks the journal writing made it really clear to Alan that the main reason for his depression and comfort eating was because he was spending too much time working and not enough time with his family. After making some changes to his work schedule he no longer needed to comfort eat and finally made good progress with his weight-loss goals.

Balancing your blood sugar can have really positive effects. It is the best way of getting rid of cravings and it often helps to reduce premenstrual problems. Along with taking regular exercise, it is also an excellent way to improve a cranky metabolism that has become sluggish due to following a succession of calorie-counting diets. Maintaining a stable blood sugar level is fundamental to this eating plan as it helps to create the ideal conditions for your body to shed excess weight. After following these guidelines for a short time you should notice that those extra pounds start to slip away because your metabolism is now starting to work very efficiently. The specific foods to eat regularly to achieve this aim are outlined in Chapter Eight (and summarized in Chapter Eleven).

chapter 5

Building the Health Pyramid

Taking steps to make sure that your blood sugar levels stabilize is an extremely important part of this weight-loss plan. However, for some people this alone is not enough. Even if they stick rigidly to an eating plan calculated to balance their blood sugar levels they will experience cravings and occasionally have the desire to overeat.

There are three reasons why this might be happening. Each is associated with a particular reason why we can be overweight or find it incredibly difficult to lose weight.

David's Problem with Wheat

David, a 35-year-old entertainer, had been yo-yo eating for years. Every few days he would have uncontrollable binges on bread, potato crisps (chips), biscuits, cookies and cakes. Once he started to eat he simply couldn't stop until everything in sight had been consumed. During such episodes he could easily eat his way through a loaf of bread, two or three packets of biscuits (cookies) and more. He also suffered from a host of digestive complaints including acid indigestion and constant bloating. His stress levels were very high due to a combination of working extremely long hours and not enjoying his work. He frequently felt exhausted and drained of energy.

As David was continually rushing from appointment to appointment, he would go for long periods without eating. When he did manage to stop for five minutes and grab something it was usually fast-releasing carbohydrate food. High levels of stress exacerbated the problem. On the face of it, David's symptoms and lifestyle pointed towards a typical blood sugar imbalance. But the extreme nature of his cravings and the type of food he satisfied these with strongly suggested that there was something else was going on. All of the clues pointed towards one major culprit, an intolerance to wheat.

To test whether we were on the right track, I suggested to David that he eliminate all sources of wheat from his diet. I also recommended steps for him to stabilize his erratic blood sugar (as described in the last chapter) and we did a bit of work to improve the condition of his digestive system, which was functioning at less than its best.

David's response to the new eating plan was dramatic. Within a week of eliminating wheat from his diet his cravings had totally disappeared. His blood sugar recovered rapidly and he started to feel much more emotionally balanced. He also had a lot more energy. David was even more amazed at the speed of his improvements than I was. He said: 'I only came to see you as a last resort, and to be quite honest I really didn't believe this would work. I've tried lots of different things in the past with no success. I'm absolutely delighted. I feel like a completely different person'.

David continued on a wheat-free diet and blood sugar balancing programme for a few months, during which time we corrected for various nutritional deficiencies and continued to stabilize and strengthen his digestive system. The improvements that he had noticed within the first week continued to build so that by the end of three months he felt much more healthy and energetic.

He felt less stressed by his work, but now that he felt stronger both mentally and physically he was taking steps towards a career change. At this point we both felt that it would be interesting to see how he would react to eating wheat again. He discovered that he could tolerate small amounts once in a while. Occasionally eating wheat now produces no ill effects and doesn't propel him into a full-blown binge.

The extent of David's cravings suggested more than a blood sugar problem and pointed strongly towards a food intolerance. A suspicion that wheat was the underlying problem was based on the fact that he satisfied his cravings and overeating primarily with wheat-based foods, but the journey to improved health required a combination of factors. He needed to follow strategies to balance his blood sugar and strengthen his digestive system as well as avoid the food that appeared to be triggering his symptoms. However, it is unlikely that David would have made such dramatic improvements or totally overcome his cravings if the wheat intolerance had not been addressed at the outset. This was because food intolerance was an underlying factor in all of the other symptoms that he was experiencing.

Levels Within the Pyramid

It is my experience from clinical practice that a person's symptoms appear to be linked together in the shape of a pyramid with distinct levels. Most symptoms can be placed within three, or possibly four, levels. At the top are the specific symptoms unique to that individual. Examples include skin problems, headaches, mild depression or aching joints. The middle levels consist of symptoms such as blood sugar imbalance and premenstrual problems. On the bottom level are factors such as a food intolerance or nutritional problems with the digestive system.

Each of these symptoms and levels are related to each other in an ascending order. Thus, the top level symptoms such as headaches might be provoked by a blood sugar imbalance which gets worse during the run-up to a period. However, both a blood sugar imbalance and premenstrual symptoms may in turn be provoked by the condition that is on the next layer down on the pyramid, such as food intolerance. In other words, working with the top or intermediate levels of the pyramid alone will only be partially successful if problems relating to the underlying, foundation level of the pyramid are not addressed.

For example, someone who is experiencing frequent headaches (assuming there is no direct medical cause) is unlikely to experience much of an improvement from just taking a herbal remedy or supplement if the headaches are linked to underlying conditions. These conditions, such as blood sugar problems and food intolerance, need to be addressed. We need to begin by working with the foundation level of the pyramid. Then we can expect to see improvements filtering up through the other levels as well. As this approach is holistic, the emotional life of the individual can also figure prominently in the symptom pyramid. Sometimes the foundation layer can be purely emotional in nature, as when relationship difficulties filter through into a host of physical symptoms. Even the best diet in the world and regular exercise are unlikely to be 100% successful if the emotional foundation to the problem is not addressed.

A Weight Loss Pyramid

The same pyramid approach can be applied to difficulties in losing weight. An example of such a pyramid might have food cravings at the top level. These, in turn, might be related to a blood sugar imbalance (intermediate level) and the problem perpetuated by a food intolerance (foundation level). Unless the problems at ground (foundation) level are addressed the blood sugar and food cravings will continue. This will result in overeating, making it impossible for the individual concerned to lose weight.

Food intolerance frequently plays a role in blood sugar problems, but it is certainly not the case that *every* blood sugar imbalance is caused by food intolerance. A large percentage of blood sugar conditions are simply related to the factors outlined in the previous chapter and will improve when corrective dietary measures are taken.

Alan's situation, which was discussed in the previous chapter, is a good example of a weight loss pyramid. His cravings for sweet foods meant that he was unable to lose weight however hard he tried to stick to a diet (top level). The intermediate level was a blood sugar imbalance which added a physical component to his craving for food. The foundation level was the stress he experienced in his job which perpetuated the blood sugar imbalance (frequent stress is a major factor in a blood sugar imbalance) and also linked directly to his need to comfort eat because of the emotional component. Alan needed to work with both a physical and an emotional strategy to break his pattern. Following a blood sugar balancing diet helped to ease the physical desire to overeat and also gave his body support to deal with the stress he was experiencing, but the main key to unlocking this vicious cycle was to re-evaluate and change the way he handled his job.

Amanda is a full-time mother with two young children. When she came to see me she told me that her weight had been steadily increasing over the past eight years. She felt that she needed to lose more than 27kg/60lb. She had tried lots of different diets, but none had produced any results. Her specific symptoms appeared to form a classic pyramid. The foundation level appeared to be a digestive imbalance which provoked a wheat intolerance (first intermediate level). This prompted a blood sugar problem (second intermediate level) which resulted in her overeating and craving foods that contained wheat (top level). She also experienced frequent panic attacks (top level). I suggested that she experiment with a wheat-free diet and also recommended ways of balancing her blood sugar and improving her digestive system.

After four weeks on this diet she returned for her second consultation. She reported that her panic attacks had practically vanished, but complained that she had not lost any weight. I was rather surprised at this as I was pretty sure that wheat intolerance was a key factor in her condition. After talking with her for a few more minutes it emerged that she had not been following a wheat-free diet for more than two days at a time.

She was going out for cake and hot chocolate with friends every other day, cooking large meals (three courses plus dessert) at home and eating biscuits (cookies) before she went to bed. The only part of the programme that she had followed was eating a few more complex carbohydrates and cutting down on caffeine. This had helped to balance her blood sugar, which was why the panic attacks had lessened. Amanda's explanation for not following the other guidelines was simply that there had been visitors staying, so she couldn't make these changes.

In Amanda's case there was a further problem at foundation level that I hadn't been aware of. This was a mental/emotional issue. Consciously she wanted to lose weight, but she was sabotaging herself on a regular basis by overeating and choosing foods that were obviously not going to support this objective. In Chapter One I stated that when there is a lack of congruency on all levels of our being it is very difficult to achieve a goal. With Amanda I suspect that there are underlying issues which create a lack of congruency. Unconsciously she is making sure that her weight remains at what she perceives as her 'psychological set point'. This doesn't make Amanda 'wrong' or 'bad'; it's simply that she needs to unravel her internal conflict if she wants to reach her goal. This will happen at the right time. She may decide that the state of congruency for her is to be satisfied with herself at her current weight. Alternatively, she may uncover some personal insights as to why she is not letting herself achieve her target.

Craving the Wrong Foods

The link between blood sugar and food intolerance is as a result of a trigger mechanism that operates when the offending food is eaten. This mechanism stimulates the body into creating an abnormally low blood sugar. This is why experiencing a drop in energy levels shortly after eating a specific food can be a signal that food intolerance is present. And, as we know, when our blood sugar is low we are likely to suffer cravings. A strange paradox of the food intolerance puzzle is that we crave the very foods we are intolerant to. No-one knows exactly why this is. Cravings like these come from physical triggers, which makes them incredibly hard to resist. What often happens is that these cravings create a cycle that perpetuates blood sugar problems, stops us from losing weight and adversely affects our overall well-being. In response to the craving, we eat the food to which we are intolerant, which triggers a low blood sugar condition, which causes us to crave more of the same food and so on.

With such a scenario, it is easy to see how weight-loss efforts could be disrupted. The best way out of this cycle is to avoid the offending food(s) completely for a short period, generally up to about four months. After this time, provided steps have been taken to improve digestive function (as we saw in Chapter Three, a weakened digestive system can be a factor in developing food intolerance), an individual can usually consume moderate amounts of the offending food without problems. Once the culprit food has been removed from the diet, cravings will normally subside quite quickly. Stick to a healthy eating plan and achieving weight-loss will be much easier.

Take a moment to consider the particular types of foods that you crave. It may be helpful to make a list of these foods and break them down into their basic ingredients and look for links between them. In David's case, his cravings were mainly for biscuits (cookies), bread and cakes. The nature of these foods, combined with his other symptoms, pointed strongly towards an intolerance to wheat. Your list will give you extremely useful information regarding your own trigger foods.

Wheat is often the main culprit when it comes to intolerance-induced cravings. Two other culprits commonly associated with cravings are sugar and yeast. Cravings associated with these foods include candy, chocolate, alcohol and yeasted breads. If these are on your list of trigger foods you will probably benefit from avoiding them for the time being.

Mood Foods

I'm sure that we have all experienced the urge to reach for a piece of cake when we are feeling a bit down or out of sorts. We generally put this desire for carbohydrates down to emotional comfort eating but there can also be a physical explanation. If specific events are causing us to feel unhappy or depressed, this type of eating is probably emotional in nature, but when we are feeling a little bit down for no apparent reason there may be a physical link involved.

Neurotransmitters are chemical messengers that travel in the bloodstream, influencing how we feel and triggering various physical processes. The neurotransmitter serotonin governs our mood. Sufficient levels of this chemical in our blood mean we feel good, but when levels fall we start to feel down. Serotonin is unique in that the amount found in the blood is related to food intake on a daily basis. When serotonin levels fall we are more likely to crave carbohydrates. The body does not use carbohydrates to make serotonin, but by eating carbohydrates we create the conditions in the body that enable it to convert a specific amino acid (a molecule of protein derived from food) into serotonin. The result is that after eating carbohydrates our mood can improve. Fortunately there are other ways of achieving the same effect, without having to resort to eating unhealthy carbohydrates such as cakes. The specific amino acid that is converted by the body to make serotonin is found in a number of foods that are nutritionally sound. If we regularly eat these foods, we are more likely to keep our serotonin levels up, and our mood high. This is particularly useful during times when we are likely to crave carbohydrates such as the run-up to a period or during the winter months when we are feeling the effects of a lack of sunshine.

Taking Positive Action

What is really exciting about this process is that we can adopt a specific eating strategy for every day that will help us to avoid craving the unhealthy refined carbohydrate foods that hamper our weight-loss efforts. If we eat a small amount of a serotonin-supporting food – a mood food snack – about half an hour before having our main meal, we are much less likely to want to eat high levels of carbohydrates then, and this will help us to reduce naturally the quantity of food that we eat. This is not just because we will feel less hungry as a result of eating the snack. Nor is it about boosting a low blood sugar (although, of course, it does this as well). It is working at an even more subtle level that influences our brain chemistry. A number of scientific studies have found that this type of eating strategy is very effective. Participants in these studies did not ask for carbohydrates like bread with their meals when they had eaten a mood food snack beforehand.

Fish not only helps the body to produce serotonin, it is also a good mood food for another reason. Oily fish such as salmon, mackerel and herring are excellent sources of specific healthy fats that work directly with the brain to improve our sense of well-being. This class of healthy fats also provides us with a hormone-like substance that helps us to lose weight. So we gain in a number of ways by making fish a regular part of our diet.

All the mood foods are strongly recommended as part of this weight loss plan as they are also high in nutritional value.

Vitamin and Mineral Deficiencies

The final factor that may be associated with cravings or overeating is being deficient in vitamins and/or minerals. If we are not getting all the nutrients that our bodies need from our food then the biochemical 'keep eating' switch can be permanently set to the 'on' position. This is the body's way of attempting to satisfy the need for these nutrients. Feeling hungry a lot of the time, even when we are eating quite large quantities of food, can be the body's way of signalling to us that something is missing from our diet. It's as if the body will keep demanding food until these nutrient requirements are met.

Eating foods that are naturally high in the particular amino acid that is a precursor to serotonin regularly will help to give your mood a boost. Many of these foods make excellent snacks. Keep them handy in the office or car so you can have a couple of mouthfuls half an hour before a meal.

- avocados
- bananas
- beans
- lentils
- chickpeas

- pumpkin and sesame seeds
- almonds and Brazil nuts
- cottage cheese
- fish
- prawns (shrimp)

Governmental agencies frequently conduct studies to assess the nutrient intake of the population. The 1996 U.S. department of Agriculture Survey of Food Intake found that 62% of people were receiving less than the minimum daily requirement for both iron and vitamin C and 67% had a low folic acid intake. About a third of the population were regularly failing to get the recommended daily amount of calcium, magnesium, zinc and vitamin E. Unfortunately the results of this study are not unique. This suggests that on average, our nutrient intake does not even meet minimum requirements, let alone providing us with the optimum levels to support our health and well-being.

It is generally believed that 'a well balanced' diet will be enough to ensure we get all the vitamins and minerals we need. However, as these studies show, achieving this is far from easy.

Deficiencies of key nutrients can sabotage our weight-loss efforts in a number of ways. First, they may trigger the urge to binge. Second, the deficiencies adversely affect the metabolic function. Metabolism requires a range of specific nutrients if it is going to perform efficiently. These include the B vitamins, vitamin C, and mineral such as zinc, magnesium, copper and iron. (You will find some examples of foods that are good sources of these essential nutrients in the next chapter.) Third, nutritional deficiencies can also be associated with persistent fluid retention. If we consume lots of foods that are high in salt and do not have much fruit and vegetables, the potassium-sodium balance can become disrupted, resulting in a tendency to retain fluid.

Little to do with Overeating

A weight problem is often unconnected with overeating. The problem is the result of several different factors, which vary from person to person. I believe that the existence of nutritional deficiencies plays a role in 99 cases out of 100. Even if you are really conscientious in keeping your food intake to a good level, nutritional deficiencies can still hamper your weight loss efforts by their negative effect on your metabolism. This is one reason why this weight-loss plan emphasizes a diet that will provide you with adequate levels of all of the key nutrients that your body needs (the other reason is that it is important to receive nutrition to keep you healthy while you are losing weight).

Chapter Eight outlines the fundamental principles of this eating plan and gives you lots of ideas for tasty foods that will provide you with an adequate intake of vitamins and minerals.

Nutritional deficiencies also arise when the body's ability to absorb the nutrition from food is impaired. You may have heard the phrase 'you are what you eat' but 'you are what you can absorb' might be more accurate. 'Artificial' vitamins and minerals, such as the calcium and iron that are added to bread, are a case in point. At a molecular level these synthetic nutrients have a different form from when they are found naturally in foods and are absorbed very poorly by our digestive systems. So even though a particular food product makes claims on the label that a serving provides you with say, 25% of your daily requirements for iron, you may in fact be absorbing as little as 10% of that amount (2.5%). The same argument applies to many of the cheaper vitamin and mineral supplements on the market, as these products tend to be based on synthetic ingredients.

If our digestive processes are not functioning at their best, not even the healthiest diet in the world will ensure we absorb all the nutrients we need. A number of factors can adversely affect the ability of our digestive system to absorb nutrients. And, if the digestive system is not working properly, intolerance can be the result. The following chapter outlines some strategies for improving the digestive system.

Building your own Pyramid

Here is a short exercise which can be quite useful in highlighting the most important areas that you need to address on your weight-loss programme. Take a blank sheet of paper and draw two columns. Head one column 'physical' and the other 'emotional'.

Under the first column list all of the physical conditions you are experiencing (or think you may be experiencing) at this time. These could include a craving for sweet foods, a blood sugar imbalance, premenstrual symptoms, digestive complaints, food intolerance and a sluggish metabolism as a result of dieting in the past. In the second column make a note of any emotional issues such as frequently feeling stressed, eating when feeling down, ambiguous feelings about losing weight and the like.

On another piece of paper draw a pyramid. Divide it lengthways into three segments. Think about how each of the factors you have listed may be linked to or influenced by another factor, then place each factor in turn into your pyramid, starting with the key factor(s) at the base (foundation level). You can place more than one factor in each level. For example, the top segment of your pyramid might include three or four items, as this layer is for the symptoms that you are experiencing, such as food cravings, bloating and fluid retention. The foundation should ideally contain only one factor, or two at the most. Once you've made an assessment of your symptoms aim to work directly with the foundation level.

When you've completed your pyramid, take a few minutes to see what it says about you. The foundation level holds the key to your personal weight-loss strategy.

chapter 6

Improving the Digestive System

Improving the functioning of the digestive system might not be the first thing that we think of when we want to lose weight. However, working with this system is of prime importance for both sorting out any food intolerance problems and to help us achieve our weight-loss goals. The digestive system has a number of important functions. First, it absorbs the nutrients we derive from food. If these nutrients are not being absorbed, either because our diet is deficient, or because the digestive system isn't working as it should, we may overeat, as explained in the previous chapter. Second, the digestive tract is a major elimination channel, helping the body to clear itself of toxins. If it is not in optimum health, its ability to remove toxins and waste products will be impaired. The liver, kidneys, lymphatic system, skin and lungs will other aspects of the body's elimination channels will have to work overtime to manage the extra level of toxins that are circulating in our system. This will cause the body to become too acidic, which will hamper our efforts to lose weight. Finally, a digestive imbalance is often the underlying cause of food intolerance. Taking a few steps to support the digestive system will help to resolve this problem and it may be possible to re-introduce small quantities of the offending food in the future.

Simple Guidelines

Improving the health of our digestive system does not require a great deal of effort or mean that we have to be incredibly fastidious about what we eat and don't eat. Big improvements can be achieved by following a few straightforward guidelines, such as regularly eating certain foods.

Digestion starts in the mouth, with the act of chewing. Food then proceeds to the stomach where specific enzymes break down protein foods. The next stage of the process happens in the small intestine and also involves the liver and the pancreas. The liver triggers the gall bladder to release bile, which starts the process of breaking down dietary fat. The pancreas releases a series of enzymes. Some of these do further work on protein foods and others break down carbohydrates and fats.

At this point the food has been converted into its basic components and these can be absorbed into the body through the walls of the small intestine. The majority of absorption happens via the small intestine although the large intestine (colon) also plays a small role. Fibre, which isn't used by the body, continues through the digestive tract along with any unnecessary waste products and is eventually eliminated from the body.

Enjoying our Food

We can do a great deal to improve the functioning of our digestive system just by taking time to chew our food properly. This doesn't mean that we have to sit at the table and chew each mouthful thirty times before we swallow, in some mechanical fashion. Instead, it means that we should eat slowly and really savour the flavour and texture of the food. When we are leading busy lives it is very easy to simply gulp food down without paying too much attention to the act of eating. Slowing down, taking time to chew each mouthful and fully experiencing the taste of what we are eating can bring us lots of benefits. Not only will we derive a great deal more pleasure from eating, but we are also likely to become more fussy about the quality and conscious of the quantity of the foods we eat.

The Taste Test

Here is a little experiment for you to try. Before you start the wheat-free part of this plan, make a bowl of plain pasta or have a slice of white bread. Take a mouthful of this food and take a minute or so to chew it thoroughly. Focus on the flavour and texture of the food. Now repeat the experiment with a mouthful of fresh, organic apple. Finally repeat the process with a mouthful of any low-calorie processed diet food. There is a vast difference between the white flour foods and the apple. The latter is a 'living food' and, as such, is bursting with flavour and texture. It is unlikely that you experienced the same abundance of taste in a mouthful of pasta or white bread. Most of the processed 'diet' foods are loaded with chemicals; these reveal themselves by leaving a strong metallic taste in the mouth.

When we rush our food, we are often unaware of the level of chemicals or the lack of taste and texture. By slowing down the whole sensory experience of eating is heightened, so we become much more conscious of the type and quality of the foods we are putting into our body.

Another benefit we get from taking the time to chew thoroughly is that we will have eaten less by the time we notice the signals from our brain that we are full. So we are less likely to overeat. Finally, chewing does more than simply break down the food into smaller, more manageable units; it also bathes the food in an enzyme which starts to digest it, so that by the time it reaches the stomach, the process can continue in an efficient manner. If the food hasn't been chewed thoroughly, the stomach finds it very difficult to work with.

The Power of Enzymes

The digestion process in the stomach and small intestine requires the correct range and quantity of digestive enzymes. These are produced by the small intestine, gall bladder and pancreas. These enzymes break down food into its component parts so that these can be absorbed via the small intestine and used by the body. There are a number of reasons why our enzyme production may not be as efficient as it should be. Frequent stress can deplete our digestive enzymes, as can drinking large amounts of coffee and tea. Smoking and alcohol consumption also has a negative effect.

Enzymes can only be produced by the body if certain vitamins and minerals are present. If we are deficient in any of these nutrients our ability to manufacture enzymes will be impaired. This can create a cycle where we are unable to produce enzymes because we lack nutrients, which means we can't digest food correctly. This in turn means that the absorption of nutrients is impaired, which leads to deficiencies that stop the body from producing enzymes and so on. Using antacid tablets on a regular basis also plays havoc with our digestive enzymes as these neutralize the enzymes in the stomach. (Indigestion may be related to a *lack* of enzymes so taking antacids only makes the situation worse.) Seeds such as pumpkin and sunflower are high in zinc which is an essential mineral for the correct functioning of these digestive enzymes.

It is also suspected that certain digestive enzymes fail to function effectively when food intolerance is present. When this stage of the process is impaired we are unable to absorb all the nutrients from food and there is a greater likelihood that problems may arise in the next stage of the digestive sequence, namely the large intestine (colon).

Proteins and Carbohydrates

Mixing proteins and carbohydrates in the same meal can disrupt the functioning of the digestive enzymes. However, protein from vegetarian sources is generally much easier to digest than meat protein. Furthermore, many vegetarian sources of protein also contain carbohydrate, and most complex carbohydrate foods also contain protein. Therefore, trying to avoid mixing proteins and carbohydrates from vegetarian sources is virtually impossible. There is some value, however, in not mixing meat sources of protein with carbohydrates. For example, a meal containing either fish or chicken can be mixed with vegetables (not potatoes) and salad, but if rice, pasta or potatoes are eaten at the same time the digestive enzymes need to work doubly hard to deal with the combination.

If you eat meat, a worthwhile strategy to improve your digestive processes and simultaneously help you to lose weight is to avoid mixing proteins and carbohydrates for your larger meals (lunch and dinner). However, you can still have a snack of nuts and seeds or 'mood foods' (which are mainly carbohydrate) 20–30 minutes before a protein meal. The main-meal suggestions on the menus provided in the Kick Start Plan on page 122 alternate between mainly-protein and mainly-carbohydrate.

It is also wise to avoid eating fruit after a large meal, especially if it contained animal sources of protein. As fruit is digested much faster than protein, eating fruit after a protein meal is likely to cause indigestion.

While it is very important to drink plenty of water every day, drinking water with a meal can dilute our digestive enzymes. Avoid drinking water 15 minutes before a meal and for at least an hour afterwards.

Foods that Support the Digestive System

If we have a food intolerance, removing the food from our diet for a period of time gives our digestive processes an opportunity to recover and allows the enzymes to start functioning correctly again. We can help this process by eating a diet which is high in alkaline-forming

WAYS OF IMPROVING THE DIGESTIVE SYSTEM

The Stomach and Small Intestine	The Colon
Eat	*Eat or drink*
• pumpkin seeds	• live yogurt
• pineapple	• F.O.S. (see below text)
• papaya	• cabbage
• sprouted seeds	• carrots
• ginger	• flax seeds
	• garlic
Avoid	• blueberries, cranberries
• mixing meat protein with carbohydrate	• black cherries
• eating fruit after large meal	• black grapes
• food to which you are intolerant	• citrus fruit (pith)
	• water
Limit	
• alcohol	
• sugar	
• processed foods	

foods such as fruits and vegetables. Some specific foods are also natural sources of enzymes. These include pineapple, papaya and sprouted seeds, such as alfalfa and mung. Cabbage is particularly healing for the small intestine and colon. Foods that contain beta carotene, (especially carrots and papaya) are also beneficial. A generous helping of home-made coleslaw, made using yogurt instead of mayonnaise, is therefore an excellent dish to add to a weight-loss plan as it is not only filling, but also supports digestive health. Ginger is a very good aid to digestion. You can either add it to foods (as in a stir-fry) or make ginger tea by chopping up a small amount of root ginger and boiling it in water for five minutes. Sweeten with a little honey, if you like.

The Colon

The colon might not be the most glamorous part of the body, but it has a number of vitally important roles to play in our overall health and well-being. It transports waste products out of the body and also synthesizes some of the B vitamins. The colon is colonized by a digestive flora (bacteria) that can either support or disrupt our well-being. In ideal circumstances about 1.4–1.8kg/3–4lb of friendly bacteria reside in the colon. These bacteria are really important for our health for a number of reasons including the assimilation of certain B vitamins and ensuring that our digestive system functions well. When there are sufficient friendly bacteria, the other types of digestive flora (which do not have such a health-promoting role) are kept at a minimum. Conversely, if there is not enough good flora, then the other types of bacteria proliferate and can cause a host of digestive problems.

The quantity and quality of these friendly bacteria is highly influenced by the type of food that we eat.

Friendly bacteria thrive when the diet includes plenty of fruit, vegetables and slow-releasing complex carbohydrates. However meat, alcohol, sugar-containing foods and acidic grains such as wheat deplete these friendly bacteria. Exposure to environmental pollutants, stress and prescription drugs can also cause disruption. Antibiotics kill bacteria but they do not discriminate between the bacteria that are causing the health problem and the friendly bacteria that live in the gut. Therefore, after a course of antibiotics, the numbers of friendly bacteria are severely reduced.

When the good bacteria are depleted, an individual is much more likely to experience digestive disorders such as leaky gut, constipation, diarrhoea, abdominal bloating and flatulence. Leaky gut, as mentioned in Chapter Three, is a condition where food molecules that should be expelled can pass through the colon wall into the bloodstream. As food intolerance is often associated with a leaky gut problem it is very important to re-establish the correct levels of these friendly bacteria. There are several simple steps that we can take to do this.

The Benefits of Bio Yogurt

We can help to repopulate the colon with friendly bacteria by eating live yogurt (also called 'bio') regularly. My personal preference is for live yogurt made from soya beans as eating soya products brings lots of additional health benefits. You could also try live yogurt from sheep's milk or goat's milk as an alternative to the dairy version. Yogurt needs to be eaten regularly for it to have any effect.

Friendly bacteria are also available in supplement form (the product is referred to as a probiotic). This provides a much higher level of good digestive flora than is obtained simply from eating yogurt.

When eating yogurt (or taking a probiotic supplement) it is useful to add fructo-oligo-saccharides (F.O.S) to your diet. This is a naturally occurring non-digestible substance derived from food that provides 'sustenance' for the friendly bacteria, making them stronger and more resilient. F.O.S is available in powdered form from good health food shops (or see the resources guide if you would like to purchase it via mail order). It is naturally sweet, but it contains no calories. You can use it instead of honey or sugar to sweeten cereals and the like. Not only will it satisfy your desire for something sweet without contributing calories, you will also get the added benefit of improvements in your digestive health. F.O.S. also occurs naturally in certain foods (see Chapter Eight). Yogurt and F.O.S. are unlikely to have a big impact if the diet still consists of high levels of meat, alcohol and refined carbohydrates, so it is also important to increase your intake of foods that support friendly bacteria, such as fruit and vegetables.

Fruit, Flax Seeds and Fibre

Other foods that can help to rectify a leaky gut problem are blueberries, black cherries, cranberries and black grapes. These contain a substance that can strengthen the gut wall. The pith from citrus fruit can also help in this respect. Flax seeds (linseeds), which you will read more about in Chapter Eight, have a very soothing and healing effect on the colon wall. You can combine all of these beneficial ingredients into a smoothie which is also an excellent blood-sugar balancing snack to have between meals.

Garlic has many beneficial properties, including its ability to improve the bacterial balance of the digestive tract. Regularly eating garlic is another worthwhile strategy.

Fruit, vegetables and complex carbohydrates also contain high levels of beneficial soluble fibre which can enhance the functioning of the digestive system. Water also plays a vital role. If we are dehydrated, we are much more likely to suffer from digestive problems such as constipation, and a simple strategy such as increasing the amount of water we drink every day can reap huge benefits in terms of our overall digestive health. It is important to remember, however that water should not be drunk with meals, or close to mealtimes.

Finally, physical activity is necessary to keep the digestive system functioning well. Taking a brisk fifteen-minute walk after eating can help us to digest and assimilate nutrition from our food.

To recap, straightforward strategies such as taking time over our food, not mixing meat proteins with carbohydrates and including plenty of fruit, vegetables, good carbohydrates and foods that are beneficial to the gut, can pay big dividends in terms of improved digestive health.

chapter 7

Get Invigorated!

The importance of our elimination channels as part of an effective weight-loss plan was highlighted in chapter two. When these systems are working properly weight-loss becomes a much easier process. The metabolism is able to perform efficiently, excess fluid can be shed easily and we are unlikely to experience the unpleasant side effects that are often associated with dieting. Supporting the functioning of these channels also has a positive effect on all aspects of our well-being. The skin becomes clearer and the hair shiny and healthier. Overall energy levels are likely to improve, bringing a sense of vibrancy and liveliness. Working with these channels doesn't require a great deal of time and effort. There are lots of simple strategies that we can adopt that will pay big dividends in terms of health and the ability to shed those extra pounds. In the previous chapter we looked at the importance of the digestive system and what we can do to improve its functioning. Here we look at the other major parts of this system, namely the liver, kidneys, lymph, skin and lungs.

The Body's Waste Disposal System

As we go about our everyday activities, the body is constantly at work, keeping itself clean and clear of toxins. Every single process that the body performs creates certain chemical by-products that need to be eliminated. These activities include repairing cells, killing viruses, metabolizing food and any type of physical movement. Even the act of breathing produces certain chemical reactions which need to be neutralized. The body has an incredibly effective 'waste disposal system" which involves the liver, kidneys, lungs, digestive system, lymphatic system and skin. Each of these provides a specific way for waste products to be eliminated, but for the process to function properly all parts need to be working well.

Whether or not the 'waste disposal system' is working properly depends on how well each part is performing and how much work the system as a whole needs to do. If any part of the system is below par and/or there is a very high level of waste products to eliminate the system can become overloaded.

We can inadvertently overload our system with toxic substances in a wide variety of ways. Chemicals added to food and drinks are prime examples. The liver is not used to dealing with these chemical compounds (they have only been used for a short time) so it has to work extra hard to break them down. Pollution in the environment, such as car exhaust fumes, cigarette smoke and abrasive household and gardening products, also contributes to our exposure. As the total exposure to toxins in our environment today is so great our elimination channels are having to work very hard to keep pace.

When a particular part of the elimination system is not functioning properly, this creates an added burden for the rest. For example, if our intestines are working sluggishly, we may become constipated. When we are unable to eliminate wastes through this channel efficiently, the other parts of the system have to work twice as hard. This puts an extra strain on the liver and lymphatic system in particular. When we are constipated we tend to feel groggy, mentally sluggish, irritable or fatigued. This is because the system has become overly acidic, due to increased level of toxins circulating in the bloodstream. These would ordinarily be removed by the liver, but when levels are unacceptably high, it is unable to process the molecules as quickly as it should.

Toxins that cannot be eliminated immediately are stored in fat cells. Fat cells make a very good storage site for potentially dangerous toxins, because they play virtually no part in the various metabolic activities of the body. Cellulite is essentially stored toxins. From a naturopathic point of view, one of the reasons why we hold on to our fat tissue, even when our calorie intake is low, is because the body is unable to deal with the added toxic load that would ensue if the toxins were released. When we lose weight and burn off fat cells the toxins they hold are released into the bloodstream. If our elimination channels are not working properly, they will not be able to withstand this increased toxic load. The body therefore makes sure that our fat cells remain on our hips so that more vital parts of the body are not put in danger.

Keeping it Alkaline

One of the key things we can do to make weight loss easier and to avoid side effects like constipation, headaches, lack of energy and dull, lifeless skin that are associated with dieting, is to keep the body in an alkaline state. The food we eat plays a big role in this respect. The body's acid-alkaline balance is adjusted throughout the day depending upon what foods we consume. Wheat, other grains and protein foods leave an acidic residue when they are metabolized. Fruit and vegetables, on the other hand, leave an alkaline residue. This doesn't mean that we should never eat protein or grains. These foods are important to our overall health and well-being. But if we balance protein and grain intake with large amounts of fruits and vegetables the body is more likely to remain alkaline. Specific advice on how to balance carbohydrates, protein and fat is given in the next chapter. Drinking sufficient water will also help the system to flush out toxins and keep elimination channels functioning well. Other substances that increase the acidity of the body are caffeine, salt, alcohol and chemicals added to foods.

The Liver and Kidneys

The liver performs a great many functions, including metabolizing food and converting it into energy or fat tissue. It also breaks down chemical wastes (in particular drugs and alcohol) which are then transported to the digestive tract for elimination. Liver function is strongly linked with the health of the digestive system. Both lack of digestive enzymes and frequent constipation create a much heavier workload for the liver, which may become unable to detoxify the system effectively.

There are a few simple steps that we can take to support liver function. Reducing our intake of both animal protein and saturated fat will help the liver to perform better. Vitamin C helps the liver to function properly so a diet rich in this nutrient is beneficial. Vitamin C is mainly found in fruit, especially guavas, kiwi fruit, berries and papaya. Sweet peppers, broccoli and red cabbage are good vegetable sources. Freshly-made juices (in particular grapefruit, and also carrot) also provide good support for the liver. A glass of hot water with the juice of half a lemon is great to have first thing in the morning to get your liver geared up for the day ahead. Physical activity of any kind is also extremely important, as this helps the liver to metabolize toxic wastes.

Silymarin is a herbal preparation, available from good health food shops, that is healing and supportive to the liver. This can be taken for short periods of time (1–2 months) while simultaneously following a diet designed to increase the alkalinity of the body.

The kidneys need plenty of fluid if they are to function at top form. Aside from drinking plenty of water, there are certain foods that can be particularly supportive of the kidneys. These include watermelon, celery, cucumber and papaya. Drinking cranberry juice can also be helpful. Cutting down on both salt and refined sugar is important as well.

The Lymphatic System

The lymphatic system has a number of vitally important tasks to perform, and plays a major role in the elimination of waste products. It consists of a series of channels (similar to veins and arteries) that circulate fluid (lymph) in a one-way direction throughout the body. The fluid acts as a carrier, allowing for any dead cells or toxins to be removed from the body via the lymph nodes. Unlike the cardiovascular system, which has the heart to pump blood around the body, the lymphatic system does not have any internal help to circulate the fluids through the system. Instead, the efficiency at which the lymph circulates depends on lifestyle. The more active we are, the better the lymph will flow, and the more efficient the removal of toxins. The more sedentary we are the harder it is for the lymph to flow, making it more difficult for toxins to be eliminated.

Supporting the System

There are two specific strategies we can adopt to support our lymphatic system. Both of these are enjoyable to do. Skin brushing can help to move the lymph, clear cellulite and improve the condition of the skin. You need a natural bristle brush, which you can purchase from a good health food shop or department store. Use the brush on dry skin. Brush each area of the body in turn, always going in a direction towards the middle of the chest by the breastbone (the location of the thymus gland, which is an important part of the lymph system). Brush up each leg from foot to thigh, up the arms from the fingers to the shoulder, up the abdomen and back, then down the top part of the chest towards the breastbone. Use a reasonably firm stroke but don't brush so hard that the skin is scratched. Be firmer on your legs and arms but adopt a gentler stroke when you are working on your abdomen. Avoid the breasts. You can spend a bit of extra time on any areas that have cellulite. It only takes a few minutes to brush the whole body.

Skin Brushing helps to move the lymph, clear cellulite and improve the condition of the skin. Do it first thing in the morning, before you get into the shower, and you'll feel invigorated, with skin that tingles, once you have finished.

Bouncing (rebounding) is great for the lymph, as well as being a good aerobic workout. You can buy a mini-trampoline from most department stores or sports shops. It doesn't cost a great deal and it will last you for years. About 5–15 minutes a day is all you need to get great benefits, but you can bounce for longer if you feel like it. Any type of physical activity will support your lymph system but bouncing is particularly good in this respect. You don't have to be extremely energetic to benefit; even gentle bouncing will have a good effect. If you're feeling more active you can play with different moves such as jumping jacks and twists. You can even bounce whilst watching your favourite TV show. Wait for at least two hours after eating, before using the bouncer.

Massage is an additional method of moving lymph. Having a massage once in a while is therefore not only very pleasurable and a great way of pampering ourselves but it is actually very good for our health as well.

Be Active

Exercise is very helpful to every part of your elimination system. It makes the liver's work of breaking down toxins much easier, it helps the digestive system to function better and it moves lymph through the system. Exercise also helps to eliminate toxins via the skin (sweating) and via the lungs (which are more active when we are moving). Finally, exercise improves the rate at which the metabolism burns up calories.

Going to the gym is great, but there are also many other ways in which we can build more physical activity into the average day. Instead of taking the lift (elevator), walk up and down the stairs. Walk on escalators or moving walkways, rather than standing still. For short journeys, leave the car at home and go on foot. When going to work, get off the bus one stop earlier and walk the rest of the way. Taking a brisk 15-minute stroll after lunch can re-energize you and clear your mind for the afternoon's activities. Jump on a bouncer while watching your favourite TV show rather than sit in an armchair.

Have Fun!

I am a great believer in having fun as much as possible. That is one of the key reasons why I emphasize that food should be fun and enjoyable, not something that we associate with a struggle. Weight loss is easier and more effective when this approach is taken. The same guideline applies to exercise. Many people embark upon an exercise plan and really battle with it because they find it boring or a chore. Often the result is that they give up after a few weeks. If we can find exercise we actually enjoy, it will be much easier to stick to.

There are plenty of options available. See what activities and classes your local sports centre or health club provides. Choose ones that sound like fun and, if you like them, go regularly. Dancing is a fantastic aerobic workout as well as an enjoyable activity. Try a belly dancing class or a salsa class so that you get some variety. Or just go out dancing at a club with friends. Weekend breaks that involve trekking or cycling in the countryside are other enjoyable ways of increasing your level of physical activity without it seeming like a chore.

If you want to give your metabolic system a good boost it is important to do some form of exercise at least every other day. This should be in a form that makes you sweat and gets your heart rate up. About 45 minutes is as long as you need. Check with your doctor if you have any health problems that might make this difficult. If you are not used to it, it can take a couple of weeks to get into the routine of exercising, but once it becomes a habit, you will find yourself relaxing and starting to enjoy yourself.

Saunas and steam baths are excellent to improve the functioning of your elimination channels as they encourage your body to sweat. A sauna or steam bath at least twice a week is both good for us and an extremely relaxing and enjoyable activity to help us to unwind at the end of a busy day. It is great for improving the condition of the skin as well.

chapter 8

Bringing the Team Players Together

In the previous chapters we met each of the key players of your weight-loss team. We are now in a position to bring these individuals together. Removing wheat from your diet for a period of time is an important part of this programme. For some people, making this adjustment to their diet can be the key to shifting some stubborn pounds or eliminating excess fluid. Eliminating wheat is only part of the picture, however. It is also important to create the conditions where it is possible for the body to lose weight easily and permanently. To achieve this goal we need to consider a number of things, including working with our metabolism, making sure we don't succumb to cravings and keeping our body in an alkaline state.

All these can be achieved by getting the right balance of carbohydrate, protein and fat in our diets and by choosing food that is highly nutritious, so that we receive all the vitamins and minerals that we need. When we get this balance right we support the metabolism and are able to shift our set point in a steady and stable fashion towards our ideal weight.

Other key players of our weight loss team are there to support the digestive system so that we are able to absorb nutrients better and can overcome any food intolerances. We also need to make sure that the liver, kidneys, lymphatic system and skin are well and eliminating waste products efficiently. When we have these five aspects in place weight loss should happen easily and be permanent.

TEAM TARGETS

- Eliminate wheat
- Support the metabolism with a healthy, balanced diet
- Keep the body alkaline
- Support the digestive system
- Help the body deal with toxins by eating the right foods, exercising and drinking plenty of water

In this chapter you will be presented with a road map to steer you through the food maze so that you have clear directions as to which foods to eat and which to avoid. Food groups have been classified into four different categories: fruits and vegetables; carbohydrates; protein and fats (see also the list provided in the appendix for specific foods in each category). I have given some suggestions regarding the number of servings to have from each group per day, but as everyone has unique dietary needs, please feel free to adjust these slightly to suit your personal circumstances. Listen to the signals your body is giving you in this respect to identify what your needs are.

Vegetables and Fruit

There is no limit on how many vegetables you may have on this plan. In fact, the more you eat the better. Vegetables are an excellent source of dietary fibre and contain high levels of vitamins and minerals. They release their energy slowly to form an important part of your blood sugar balancing strategy. In terms of the acid-alkali balance, all vegetables will support your body's move towards an alkaline state, when it will be much easier for you to lose excess weight.

In summer months aim to eat vegetables in their raw state. A plate of crudités (carrots, celery, cucumber, broccoli, peppers) with some guacamole or hummus is very filling and provides your body with a range of important nutrients. Have a bowl of corn chips or some baked potato skins if you want to make the snack a bit more substantial. A large raw salad with avocado and perhaps a protein food such as a tuna steak provides an excellent evening meal. In the winter months you can get your vegetable intake from stews, soups and stir-fries. When cooking vegetables, steam them or boil them as this reduces the amount of nutrient loss.

It takes a bit of time to eat a plate full of vegetables or a bowl of salad. As mentioned earlier, taking your time over a meal can increase the satisfaction that you get from eating. It also has an important psychological element as you are less likely to feel deprived when you have given yourself the time to sit down and eat a full plate of food. Adding a little bit of olive oil and lemon or a tablespoon of vinaigrette dressing to your salad is definitely recommended (see below).

Fruit is also a very important part of this plan. Most fruit is very good at helping to support a stable blood sugar. Anti-oxidant vitamins are found in many fruits. And, like vegetables, fruit leaves an alkaline residue after being metabolized. Canned and frozen fruit is not as good as fresh and may also contain added sugar. Dried fruit should be eaten in moderation only as it is high in sugar. An easy way of adding more fruit to your diet is to make a fresh fruit salad. (A combination of melon, papaya, kiwi fruit, strawberry, pineapple and passion fruit is my favourite.) This will keep fresh in the refrigerator for about three days. You can have a bowl between meals or add a couple of spoonfuls to your breakfast cereal. Fruit smoothies are also excellent. Experiment with different combinations of fruits. I particularly like watermelon with strawberries, blueberries and kiwi fruit. Blend a handful of berries with a large slice of melon and enough water to create the correct consistency. If you add some live yogurt and some ground nuts and seeds, you will have a substantial meal-in-a-glass that makes a quick breakfast or afternoon snack.

Keep fruit at work as a snack for when you get peckish. As fruit is digested quickly it is best to eat it either before a meal or at least two hours after, especially if the meal contained meat. Cut down on raw fruits during the winter months if you live in a part of the world that gets really cold and damp. Increase your vegetable intake to compensate.

Fruit and vegetables are very easy to digest. If you have difficulty with these foods it suggests that your digestive system could do with a little bit of support. Once you have incorporated some of the suggestions from Chapter Six and removed from your diet any foods to which you are intolerant you should expect to see an improvement in your digestion. You may not be used to eating a diet high in fruit and vegetables. If this is the case, please don't be put off by the recommendation to make these foods a big part of your diet. You don't have to make a dramatic shift overnight. Start by increasing your intake slowly, perhaps by making vegetables a large part of two meals for the first week, then three meals for the next week and so on. Experiment with new recipes that use different herbs and flavours. Once you get accustomed to these foods you will find that they really are very tasty.

Carbohydrates

Refined carbohydrates, which are present in most wheat-containing foods and anything that is processed and/or high in sugar, can definitely add inches to our hips. They fail to support our blood sugar balance and they confuse our metabolism. These types of foods are generally devoid of nutritional value and high in fat as well. So carbohydrates like these are best avoided by anyone who wants to lose weight and improve their overall health.

Complex carbohydrates, on the other hand, totally support our weight-loss efforts. They are the body's favourite source of energy and foods that are high in complex carbohydrates should form a crucial part of your diet if you want to lose weight. These foods are the key to keeping your blood sugar stable, avoiding cravings and making sure that your metabolism functions optimally. Eat them regularly and you should notice that you have lots more energy and do not experience the fatigue and grogginess that often accompanies dieting.

There is a long list of complex carbohydrates to choose from. Vegetables and fruit contain carbohydrates. Grains, beans and legumes are excellent complex carbohydrates. They are packed with nutrients and are also very enjoyable to eat. Breakfast grains worth trying include millet flakes, buckwheat, oats, oat bran and barley flakes. Beans and peas make excellent additions to salads in the summer or can be added to stews and soups in the winter. Most supermarkets carry a wide range of beans and peas, including kidney, pinto, butter and lima beans and chickpeas. The canned beans are as good as the dry ones, so if time is short you don't need to worry about soaking them overnight. It is important, however, to rinse canned beans and chickpeas thoroughly under the cold water tap to remove any salt. Beans and peas, tossed in a vinaigrette dressing with a few added herbs work very well as a quick snack food or as part of a summer lunch. The mixture will stay fresh in the fridge for several days.

Complex carbohydrates to have with main meals include: brown rice, rice noodles (good in a stir-fry), lentils or potatoes (with skins). All of these make tasty alternatives to the refined carbohydrates found in pasta. Grains and beans take only a short while to cook, so you don't need to stand over a hot stove for hours to make a healthy evening meal.

Some of my clients look very sceptical when I suggest they eat these particular foods, but it is usually the case that they find the addition of these new ingredients to their diet very palatable. Most continue to eat these foods after their health problem has improved or when they have reached their ideal weight. So, if these foods are not your usual fare, keep an open mind and experiment with some of the recipes provided by Antoinette.

Good Sources of Fibre

Complex carbohydrates are very filling which means that you don't need to eat large portions to feel satisfied. They are slow-releasing, so you will feel full between meals as well, but not bloated or sluggish. These foods are gentle on the digestive system so you shouldn't experience these unpleasant side effects.

Complex carbohydrates are also excellent sources of soluble fibre, which will help to keep the digestive system functioning at top form. They are also a very good source of the vitamins and minerals we need to keep our metabolism working well.

The only drawback to these carbohydrates is that they are acid-forming. Wheat is one of the worst offenders in this respect as it is highly acidic, but most of the other grains are slightly acidic. Combining carbohydrates with alkali-forming fruits and vegetables will help reduce this impact.

Three to four servings of complex carbohydrates a day is all that is needed to obtain the benefit of these foods. As an example, three servings might consist of a bowl of wheat-free muesli for breakfast, mixed beans with a green salad for lunch, and a portion of brown rice with stir-fried vegetables and tofu for dinner. A handful of nuts and seeds (which are both carbohydrate and protein) can be added as snacks between meals.

Protein

One of the main functions of protein foods is to provide the raw materials the body needs to rebuild and repair itself. For effective weight loss we need to get the right balance of protein in our diet. Protein is important, but too much is potentially damaging. Protein foods are acidic which means they create an acidic environment within the body. This helps to explain why people who go on a high-protein, low carbohydrate diet often feel tired and anxious. Too much protein in the diet is also associated with an increased risk of osteoporosis (brittle bones).

The type of protein that we choose is also a very important consideration. Some protein foods (such as cheese and meat) are very high in saturated fat, which is something we can do without. If you do eat meat, it is best to choose cuts that are very lean. Trim off any fat and cook it in such a way that any excess fat drains out.

Better sources of protein are found in foods such as oily fish (which contains some important fats that help the metabolism) and vegetarian protein sources such as soya. Tofu, which is a curd made from soya beans, makes a great addition to stir-fries, for instance. Soya foods are extremely good for our overall health for a great number of reasons, so it is an excellent idea to incorporate these into your diet. Tofu (bean curd) is a very versatile food that is easy to cook. Or try live soya yogurt (sold as Yofu) and soy milk in cooking.

Quinoa is another food that you might like to try. It is one of the best sources of protein available, containing more protein weight-for-weight than steak, but is virtually fat free. Quinoa is a grain that is cooked in the same way as rice but which only needs to be boiled for about 10 minutes. Mix it with other grains and add some spices to improve the flavour. Most health food shops stock it. Another fantastic source of low-fat protein that you can experiment with is sprouted beans and seeds, such as mung beans, alfalfa and chickpeas. Sprouts are a very good source of protein and contain a whole range of enzymes that are great for the digestive system. They are also alkaline. You can sprout your own beans, but this is somewhat time-consuming. Most health food shops stock a good range and they are very inexpensive. Add them to salads or mix them into soups.

As part of your weight loss plan you may want to avoid mixing certain protein foods with carbohydrate. This strategy can speed up weight loss and is beneficial for the digestive system, but it is only really worthwhile to do this when you are eating meat or fish. Vegetarian sources of protein such as soya foods, quinoa and sprouts generally mix well with complex carbohydrates, and most of the foods listed in the carbohydrate section are sources of protein anyway. For example, mixing rice and lentils gives you a complete protein, which means that it provides all the essential amino acids as well as a complex carbohydrate meal. A strategy you might like to try for main meals is to alternate the protein/vegetable combination with the carbohydrate/vegetable combinations. For instance, you could have grilled (broiled) salmon with vegetables and salad (no potato) as your protein meal and ratatouille with mixed beans and rice as your carbohydrate meal. The menu plans later in this book loosely follow this strategy of separating protein and carbohydrates for lunch and dinner.

Yogurt (preferably live), cottage cheese and eggs are other worthwhile sources of protein. Nuts such as almonds, walnuts and brazils also provide protein and give you a balanced source of calcium and magnesium. Between two to three servings a day of protein is all that most people need. This might consist of a tub of soya yogurt with fruit for breakfast, a baked potato with cottage cheese and salad for lunch and a tuna steak with steamed vegetables, rice and salad for dinner.

Fats: the Good, the Bad and the Ugly

Many people attempt to avoid fats when they are on a diet because fats have a higher level of calories per gram than either protein or carbohydrates. Saturated fats should definitely be reduced, as these can have a negative impact on our health and our weight-loss efforts. However, certain other fats are essential for keeping our metabolic rate functioning effectively. Without a good intake of these fats, the metabolism can become sluggish, which will make weight loss harder than it needs to be.

Saturated fats are found in cheese, meat, milk, butter and eggs (and foods that contain one or more of these ingredients, such as chocolate). Saturated fats are the 'bad fats' that are linked to high cholesterol and heart disease. These are the fats that it is important to cut down on; they just provide us with empty calories and do little to support overall health. The average British or North American diet contains far too much saturated fat and is deficient in the other healthier types of fat.

Simple steps such as substituting cottage cheese for regular cheese, using soya milk instead of cow's milk and choosing fish rather than meat are easy ways of reducing your saturated fat intake. Choosing to grill (broil) or bake instead of frying is also important. If you are in the habit of having meat every day, try switching to either fish or vegetarian meals for at least three evenings a week. Although they are a source of saturated fat, eggs are in all other respects a good food. As long as they are not fried, it is fine to eat them about three times a week.

Essential fats are classified into two types: omega-3 and omega-6. Nuts, seeds and vegetable oils provide varying proportions (depending on the specific food) of both omega-3 and omega-6, while oily fish is an excellent source of omega-3. Both omega-3 and omega-6 essential fats are necessary for the body in a number of ways. They are important for the proper functioning of the reproductive system, the immune system and the brain. If skin and hair are to look really healthy and glowing, we need to have a good supply of these essential fats. In addition, omega-3 fats can reduce the risk of arthritis, heart disease and certain cancers.

The Role of Omega-3 Fats

When it comes to weight loss, omega-3 essential fatty acids are particularly interesting and can help in two very important ways. First, they stimulate the metabolism, which improves the rate at which we can lose weight. A recent scientific study from the University of Western Australia compared two groups of people who were trying to lose weight. Both groups controlled their calorie intake but one group was asked to base one meal a day on fish, which was high in omega-3 fatty acids. The people who ate fish every day lost significantly more weight than the group who were just controlling calories. Several other studies have produced similar findings.

Omega-3s are also good for the brain and can improve the mood. A craving for carbohydrate, especially refined carbohydrate, often happens when an individual feels depressed. Although eating carbohydrates can lift the spirits in the short term, this but won't help with our weight-loss efforts, so a better solution is to regularly eat foods that are high in omega-3s. This will improve our mood generally, making us less liable to experience cravings. Try to include a source of omega-3 fats in your diet every day. This will prove particularly useful if you feel that your metabolism is sluggish and could do with a boost.

The best source of omega-3 is oily fish such as cod, haddock, tuna, salmon, mackerel and plaice (flounder). Try to eat fish at least three times a week. If you don't like fish or you are a vegetarian you can obtain your omega-3s from flax seeds (linseeds). Even if you do eat fish it is worth making flax seeds (linseeds) a normal part of your daily diet, so that you get a daily intake of these important fats, either as seeds or as oil. One large tablespoon every day of either is all you need. Other sources of omega-3 for vegetarians are soya beans and walnuts.

When using flax seeds (linseeds) either soak them overnight in a little water or grind them to a powder in a coffee grinder. Soaking or grinding makes the seeds easier to digest and absorb. You can add the ground or soaked seeds (or the oil) to your breakfast cereal, or eat them with yogurt. They make a great addition to a fruit smoothie. Store both the seeds and the oil in the refrigerator as they spoil easily. Only grind the seeds as you use them. Flax seeds (linseeds) are also very soothing and healing for the digestive system, so this is another good reason for eating them regularly. You can also purchase omega-3 fish oils in tablet form (but note that cod liver oil is not the same as an omega-3 supplement).

Omega-6

During the last 30 years or so the amount of omega-6 fats in our daily diet has increased dramatically. Vegetable oils are now commonly used in baking (cakes, pastries, biscuits, cookies) and most people buy low-fat spreads or margarine instead of butter. The increased consumption of these fats means that the ratio of omega-6 to omega-3 is far more than it should be. Furthermore, many of the omega-6 fats that we consume are hydrogenated fats (also called trans-fatty acids). These fats are frequently used in processed foods and are also found in margarine and low-fat spreads. Hydrogenated fats are made by a chemical process, which involves heating an oil (such as sunflower oil) and converting it into a solid (such as sunflower spread). During the process the molecular structure of the oil changes. In its new molecular form, the solid fat cannot be utilized by the body in the same way that the original oil could. Further, hydrogenated fats block the uptake of 'good' fats such as omega-3 or healthy (unhydrogenated) omega-6. In other words, having too many hydrogenated fats can produce a deficiency of omega-3 and omega-6 even if sources of these essential fats are eaten regularly. Hydrogenated fats have been associated with other health problems as well, so it is sensible to avoid them.

The optimum ratio of omega-6 to omega-3 is 1:1. One tablespoon of

OPTIMUM DAILY SERVINGS FOR EACH FOOD GROUP

Fruits and Vegetables

Eat as much as you like of these, when you are physically peckish.

- apples
- berries (all)
- broccoli
- cabbage
- carrots
- melon

Complex Carbohydrates

3–4 servings

- wheat-free muesli
- beans
- chickpeas, hummus
- brown rice
- lentils
- nuts (almonds, brazils, hazelnuts)

Protein

2–3 servings

- oily fish
- soya products
- live yogurt
- quinoa
- cottage cheese
- eggs

Lean Meat

- chicken

Fat

1–2 servings

- flax seeds
- pumpkin seeds
- sunflower seeds
- oily fish (salmon, cod, mackerel)
- sunflower oil
- sesame oil
- cold-pressed olive oil

Fluid

- Drink at least 1.5 litres, 50fl oz, 1½ quarts, but don't drink water immediately before, during or within 1 hour of eating a meal.
- Water (mineral or filtered)
- Freshly prepared juices
- Herb teas

flax oil or seeds (linseeds) every day, plus eating oily fish at least three times a week will provide ample omega-3.

We can get adequate amounts of omega-6 from eating a handful of other seeds (such as pumpkin, sunflower and sesame) each day plus one tablespoon of cold-pressed oil (safflower, sesame, sunflower) on salad or drizzled on a baked potato or grilled vegetables.

Hydrogenated fats must be avoided as much as possible. Look at the label on any food you buy; and if the words 'hydrogenated' appear on the list of ingredients, put it back on the shelf. This includes most low-fat spreads and margarine. When you are having toast or sandwiches, either use a scraping of butter or get used to eating them without added fat.

Avoid using vegetable oils for stir-frying as heat damages them. Use olive oil instead, as it is less vulnerable to heat damage. When stir-frying, heat the wok first, then add a bare trickle of olive oil just below the rim. You may be surprised to discover how little you need. The oil will run down the sides of the hot pan and provide a very thin coating. Add the food to be stir-fried, toss it constantly, and add a little water if necessary.

Juices

An essential part of this plan is to drink at least 1.5 litres, 50fl oz, 1½ quarts of water per day. This can be either bottled water or tap water that has been filtered. Still water is better than carbonated.

Freshly prepared vegetable juices are fantastic for your whole system. They contain high levels of nutrients, a number of enzymes, and help to keep your system alkaline. A juice extractor is a worthwhile investment. It is relatively inexpensive and will last for years. You can extract the juice from virtually any vegetable. Carrot is very tasty on its own and makes an excellent base to mix with other juices. Some good combinations to try are carrot and apple or carrot and celery. You can also juice cucumber, raw beetroot (beets), parsley, lettuce and peppers. Experiment to see which combinations you like best. Having one glass of vegetable juice daily is a very good addition to your weight-loss plan. Carrot juice, however, is fast-releasing so either drink it with a meal or have two or three small glasses throughout the day rather than one large glass. Fresh vegetable juices should not be stored in the refrigerator; they need to be drunk as soon as they are pressed as the vitamin and enzyme content is lost very quickly. Try not to drink water with meals. If you are eating out at a restaurant then you will probably want to drink some water or juice, because it is part of the social situation, but try to avoid this when you are at home or at work. You can have a glass of water 15 minutes before a meal but leave about an hour after eating before you drink water again. This will help your stomach's digestive juices to breakdown the food properly. It's okay to drink water with snacks between meals.

Foods to Avoid

Apart from wheat, which has already been discussed at length, there are a few other foods that you should be wary of. These include anything that is highly refined or processed as it is likely to be high in fat, full of preservatives and additives and devoid of nutrients. Anything that contains refined sugar should also be avoided as much as possible. This doesn't mean that you can never have an ice-cream or a piece of chocolate. You can, but if you are committed to your weight loss goal these foods really need to be kept to a minimum. Low calorie 'diet' versions are not a better option, as these contain high levels of artificial ingredients and chemicals.

Try having a piece of fresh fruit or a small portion of dried fruit if you really fancy something sweet. If you do eat some chocolate, have it after a complex carbohydrate meal so that it will not disrupt your blood sugar balance. Foods that contain added salt can aggravate fluid retention, so these are best avoided. Drinks that contain caffeine disrupt blood sugar balance so should be kept to a minimum. Alcohol is a source of refined sugar that also depletes nutrients from the body, especially the B vitamins and fatty acids, which are essential to the functioning of your metabolism. A glass of wine with your main meal once in a while is okay.

Avoiding the Unconscious State

I've noticed that people occasionally fall into what I've called an unconscious state when it comes to eating. This is not literally becoming unconscious, but it's a state where we are unaware of certain things that we are doing. I've certainly done this myself from time to time and have observed friends doing the same thing. It seems to happen when we are preoccupied. We might be worrying about a teenage daughter's exam results or wondering whether we will get a promotion at work and before we know it foods that we were trying to avoid have somehow miraculously been eaten! It's the same type of situation as when we are driving to a new destination but suddenly realise that we have gone the wrong way. Instead of following the planned route, we've switched off and gone into auto-pilot and are heading for shops, or wherever else we would normally be going at this time.

This sort of thing can happen all too easily when we are preparing food for the family. Here's a typical scenario. Anna is making a birthday cake while chatting to her neighbour, who has dropped in for tea. She's so engrossed in hearing the local gossip that she doesn't notice that she's been dipping into the cake mixture for the past five minutes.

A similar situation might arise when you are invited to a friend's house for dinner. You're enjoying the company and having a lot of fun, but didn't notice that your hosts topped up your plate with a second helping and your glass with yet more wine.

When we are comfort eating for emotional reasons we're often unaware of just how much we are consuming, because our minds are elsewhere. It is only when we realise that the biscuit packet is empty that we stop and think 'Gosh, I didn't realise I had eaten so much!'

You don't have to be on your guard every second of the day to avoid this type of problem. That approach would be unnecessarily stressful and could put your efforts at weight-loss back into the struggle category again. All that is really needed is increased awareness. Accept that this sort of thing happens, be aware of times that might be particularly tricky for you, then pre-empt the problem by focussing on the goal you want to achieve.

One way of doing this is to bring the image of yourself at your ideal weight (or the weight where you still feel congruent) into your mind's eye. This will shift your mental and emotional focus into the pleasure of achieving your goal, which will naturally reduce the 'unconscious' desire to eat foods you don't really want. This can be an excellent strategy to use when you know you are going out to a place where there will be a temptation to eat foods that contain wheat or which are high in fat or sugar. Mentally prepare in advance by calling up your TV screen image. Then, when your aunt offers you a large slice of the cake she has just baked you will be able to say, kindly but firmly: 'No thank you'.

Specific Foods that Support your Metabolism

Metabolism requires a range of nutrients including many of the B vitamins, zinc, magnesium, iron and vitamin C. You will get adequate levels of the B vitamins from many of the foods listed above including seeds, nuts, chicken and fish. Vitamin C is found mainly in fruit and in certain vegetables such as peppers and broccoli. Iron is more readily absorbed in the presence of vitamin C. Sources of iron include eggs, liver, shellfish and green vegetables. Iron and zinc compete for absorption so try and eat foods containing these minerals at separate meals. Zinc is found in oysters, shellfish, meat and popcorn (plain). Good sources of magnesium are almonds, hazelnuts, seaweed, dried apricots and prawns (shrimp). Seeds (pumpkin, sunflower, sesame) provide you with nearly everything you need to keep your metabolism functioning on top form, including the B vitamins, zinc, magnesium and essential fatty acids. This is why they are such excellent foods to eat regularly on your weight-loss plan. In addition, nuts and seeds (particularly sunflower and sesame seeds and almonds) also provide good quantities of vitamin E which is a vital nutrient to ensure proper thyroid function. Oily fish and flax seeds (linseeds) are the main sources of metabolism-stimulating omega-3.

Specific Foods to Help with Fluid Retention

Foods that can help to reduce fluid retention include watermelon, celery, fresh parsley and cucumber. Watermelon can be blended with another soft fruit in a mixer to make a refreshing smoothie. Include the seeds. Cranberry is a good tonic for the kidneys. Cucumber and parsley (just a handful) can be passed through a juice extractor with a small amount of carrot juice added for taste. It's also important to avoid salt, sugar and anything that contains caffeine.

Specific Foods to Support the Digestive System

The digestive system needs vitamin B6 and zinc plus certain enzymes to function effectively. Source of zinc have been listed above. Vitamin B6 is found in corn cereal, sesame seeds, hazelnuts and lentils. Enzymes can be found in fresh fruit, especially pineapples and papaya. Sprouted seeds (alfalfa, mung) are also an excellent source of enzymes. Blueberries, black grapes and cranberries contain specific compounds that can help to strengthen the gut wall. Live yogurt, which contains friendly bacteria, is important for the colon. Asparagus, cabbage and broccoli naturally contain F.O.S. (fructo-oligo-saccharides – discussed in chapter six) which support the growth of friendly bacteria in the colon. Flax seeds (linseeds) are very healing for the colon. Ginger is an all-round tonic for the digestive system.

Specific Foods that Support Stable Blood Sugar Levels

To maintain a stable blood sugar we need certain B vitamins and the minerals chromium and zinc. Good sources of chromium are prunes, asparagus, raisins and mushrooms, although mushrooms should be avoided if you have a craving foods that contain yeast. The specific B vitamins that can enhance blood sugar can be found in corn cereal, chicken, seaweed and tuna. Nuts and seeds are also very good for stabilizing blood sugar. The most important part of blood sugar control is to eat complex carbohydrate foods regularly throughout the day and avoid refined carbohydrates and stimulants.

chapter 9

Becoming Wheat Free

This chapter provides practical advice regarding what to expect from, and how to adapt to, a wheat-free diet. To help you to make this adjustment I have provided you with lots of guidelines that will make the process as pain-free and easy as possible. Eating a diet without wheat really isn't difficult, provided you spend a little time preparing for the transition and planning your daily menus. It isn't necessary to go overboard with planning, as this would be both restrictive and time-consuming, but some forethought, so that you avoid potential problems, is very useful. Following a wheat-free diet should not mean that you feel deprived or that eating and meal planning has become a major chore. There are lots of wheat-free alternative foods available, including breads and wheat-free pastas.

A Wheat-free Trial

Five weeks is generally long enough to assess the difference a wheat-free diet can make to your weight and overall well-being. View this five-week period as if you were conducting a scientific experiment. To get clear results you need to avoid wheat completely. Having even a small amount every few days or so would prevent your body from making the changes that could occur if wheat were avoided completely.

Having said that, it is important not to get obsessive about the whole thing. There is not much point in worrying every time you sit down to a meal that it might contain a few grains of wheat. That approach would just cause you unnecessary stress. Instead, you simply need to make informed choices on what you eat.

Some manufactured foods contain a very small amount of wheat. This includes some brands of soy sauce. If you order a stir-fry in a restaurant, a plateful will probably contain about a tablespoon or so of soy sauce, which in turn will contain a minuscule amount of wheat. For most people, having such a tiny amount would neither spoil the wheat-free trial nor cause an adverse reaction. However, anyone suffering from Coeliac disease must be scrupulous in avoiding wheat and other gluten grains. Soy sauce is also fermented, which means that the trace amount of wheat is not in its original form.

So please do keep things in perspective. Eating a biscuit or cookie every other day would interfere with the trial, but an occasional dash of soy sauce is unlikely to invalidate the process. Wheat-free soy sauce is available in the shops, so you can use this version at home.

The four-week trial period is a good opportunity for you to experiment with a whole range of new foods. There are so many to choose from that you need never feel you are restricting yourself. Nearly everyone I know who has tried a wheat-free diet has commented on how much they enjoyed the variety and taste of foods that were formerly unfamiliar, and in most cases, they continued to eat them regularly, even after their intolerance to wheat had cleared up.

What to Expect

The reactions to removing wheat do vary from person to person. Some people notice an improvement in their overall health and well-being within a very short period, often within three to four days. For others, it can be a few weeks before any changes are evident. Digestive problems and bloating tend to be the first symptoms to improve.

The speed at which weight loss occurs is also unique to the individual. Keith, a stockbroker, lost 4.5kg/10lb during the first week when he removed wheat from his diet. He went on to lose another 3.6kg/8lb during the following four weeks – which brought him to his ideal weight.

Samantha, a sales executive, had a different experience. She lost a steady 900g/2lb a week over a period of a few months. The majority of the weight that Keith lost during the first week was excess fluid. Not everyone will lose excess fluid so rapidly; for some people the process takes a bit longer.

A Permanent Solution

The aim of this programme is for you to achieve permanent weight loss rather than a quick-fix drop of a few pounds followed by a rebound. To reset your body's set point to a permanently lower level it is best to lose weight at a steady pace. A weight loss in the region of 450g–1.4kg/1–3lb a week is about right. Any weight you lose beyond this amount is probably excess fluid. If you cut your calorie intake significantly (which is not a part of this programme) you will also lose muscle tissue, which is something that should be avoided.

Some people (but not everyone) find that when wheat is removed from their diet there is an initial negative reaction. This usually occurs during the first three to four days. Common reactions are feeling tired or sleepy, being unable to concentrate, feeling a little bit 'spacey' or getting a headache. In addition, current health symptoms can flare up and become more troublesome. Symptoms such as tiredness and headaches generally clear up within a few days and the health symptoms associated with wheat intolerance start to subside at this point as well. Paradoxically, experiencing this reaction should be viewed as a positive sign, because it provides some evidence that an intolerance to wheat is present. In other words, it's a signal that removing wheat is probably going to be beneficial in the longer term.

When you have been following a wheat-free diet for about two weeks your body will have become highly sensitized to the grain, so if you have a meal that contains wheat at this point, you may experience an adverse reaction. This is likely to be an exaggerated version of the initial reaction that occurred in the first few days. It usually consists of a general sense of feeling unwell, accompanied by a recurrence of other health symptoms, especially digestive complaints. This sensitization peaks around two weeks after wheat is eliminated but usually subsides after that time. Therefore, it is particularly important to avoid eating wheat at this point. If you do inadvertently consume wheat and experience an adverse reaction, the best thing to do is to drink plenty of water and give yourself time to rest. Two grams of vitamin C (with food) is often helpful as is drinking some bicarbonate of soda mixed with a glass of water, on an empty stomach. The reaction normally passes within 24–48 hours.

After Five Weeks

When you have completed five weeks of a wheat-free diet, have another look at the wheat intolerance questionnaire on page 38 to assess the changes in your well-being. Some of these changes might be quite profound (such as a digestive complaint that has been with you for years suddenly clearing up) while others might be more subtle. Subtler changes include a general sense of having more energy, feeling more positive or noticing that your thinking processes are much clearer. Any changes in bloating or fluid retention (in addition to weight loss) are also significant.

If you have experienced an improvement in both health symptoms and your general sense of well-being, this provides good evidence that you may indeed be intolerant to wheat. At this point you have two options. You can either simply continue on the wheat-free plan for the medium term, without trying to find out what would happen if you reintroduced wheat, or you can test your reaction to reintroducing wheat at this point. To do this, have a meal containing wheat, such as a bowl of pasta or a couple of slices of bread, and monitor your reactions for the next 48 hours. Pay particular attention to any drop in energy levels, feelings of fatigue or any mood changes that may occur within the first few hours after a meal, and whether any of the health symptoms that cleared up while you were wheat-free return over the next couple of days, especially digestive symptoms such as bloating or digestive discomfort. If you experience any of these conditions when you reintroduce wheat, it may be worthwhile for you to return to a wheat-free diet for a little longer.

The main reason for undertaking this test is to clarify whether the changes you have experienced are directly linked to wheat. The downside is that you may experience a recurrence of health problems for a couple of days, which can be unpleasant. Many people prefer to skip this reintroduction and continue on a wheat-free diet for a bit longer, as they don't want to disrupt the improvements in their well-being that have already occurred.

For most people, continuing on a wheat-free diet for another two or three months, while simultaneously taking steps to improve the digestive system and overall health, is sufficient to overcome an intolerance, although there are some individuals for whom the process takes longer. After this time, moderate amounts of foods containing wheat are normally tolerated without too many difficulties.

Preparation & Planning

To make the transition to a wheat-free diet as easy as possible it is wise to do some preparation in advance. Fix a date in your diary for starting the wheat-free phase. A Saturday or Sunday is usually best as this gives you a day or two to get into the routine before you go back to work. Familiarize yourself with the list of foods that contain wheat in the appendix so that you know what to avoid. Have a shopping trip the week before to stock up on the wheat-free products that you would like to try.

When embarking on a wheat-free diet, most people instinctively turn to substitutes for the foods with which they are most familiar, so top of the list are alternative forms of pasta, bread and crispbreads. However, a better approach is to shift your mind-set and experiment with some new foods and menus. It is good that options such as wheat-free bread are available, but if you rely on these foods, you will be perpetrating old eating patterns. For example, you may have become accustomed to having a sandwich for lunch, so think this is the only option. Buying wheat-free bread keeps you stuck in the routine and stop you trying the multitude of quick and tasty alternative meals. Keep wheat-free bread as an occasional option.

Stocking Up

The shopping list in the appendix can give you some ideas regarding the different types of grain, pulses, flours and seeds available. There is no need to buy everything on the list; simply purchase one or two items from each category so that you have a good selection of wheat-free foods to eat. Also stock up with plenty of fresh fruits and vegetables. Make one of your kitchen cupboards a wheat-free zone.

The key to making this work easily and effectively is to plan ahead. You need to plan your meals around your particular lifestyle and requirements. Breakfast should pose absolutely no problems as there are a tremendous number of wheat-free meals to choose from. The evening meal will also be pretty straightforward as there are endless choices to be had, either at home or when eating out. Lunch may well be often the trickiest meal, especially if you are away from home. There are not that many healthy and quick wheat-free lunchtime snacks on offer, especially to buy. The local sandwich shop or the on-site restaurant at work is unlikely to have a vast range of wheat-free options. So the best solution is to carry suitable food with you.

If you are at home with children you will need to adopt different strategies to someone who lives alone and works full time. Your children and partner will probably continue to eat foods that contain wheat, so you need to be quite disciplined in keeping your wheat-free foods in a separate place and not inadvertently taking a few mouthfuls of anything of theirs that contains wheat. When you go out with the children, say to a lunchtime birthday party where the food is likely to consist of lots of wheat-rich products, take something with you that you can eat. This strategy does require forward planning and involves extra preparation time but the effort will be worthwhile. Otherwise you can be caught in a situation where you are incredibly hungry with nothing except wheat-containing foods available.

If you know your schedule you can plan your menus in advance. This will cut down on the preparation time involved. The recipes in this book include lots of dishes like Three Bean Salad and Smoked Haddock and Sweetcorn Chowder, which can be prepared ahead and which will stay fresh in the refrigerator for a few days.

Keep a selection of healthy nibbles at your workplace. A bag full of nuts and seeds is particularly important, as you should aim to eat a handful of these every day, between meals. Good foods to keep in the refrigerator at work are tubs of hummus and/or guacamole, some yogurt, cottage cheese, some carrot and celery sticks and a bottle of mineral water. A basket of fresh fruit, a packet of wheat-free crispbreads and a selection of herbal teas will round off the selection nicely. You can keep non-perishable items in the car, too. They will come in very handy if you are out on the road a lot or if you are a busy mum or dad ferrying children from one activity to another. It will save you from being tempted to grab a sandwich from a service station when you are feeling peckish. If you regularly travel away from home and stay overnight in a hotel, it is also useful to keep a bag of wheat-free muesli in the car, as hotels usually only give you a choice of cereals that contain wheat for breakfast or offer you unhealthy options like eggs and bacon.

Reading Labels

Lots of foods contain added wheat, so it is essential to check labels to make sure that you are not eating this grain inadvertently. Rye crispbread, for example, usually contains both wheat and rye. To get totally wheat-free crispbread you need to pay a visit to a health food shop (Ryvita Original is wheat free). Common foods that contain added wheat are soup, gravy, pasta sauce, sausages and canned meats. If the ingredients label states 'starch' or 'modified starch' then this may be from a wheat source. 'Maize starch' is okay, as this is derived from corn. Getting into the habit of reading the label of ingredients on foods when you do your shopping is worthwhile, even though it does take a bit longer.

Cooking for the Family

Following a wheat-free plan at the same time as cooking for your family or partner need not cause problems. Breakfast is very simple as your wheat-free meal should not conflict with anything your family currently eats. Lunch is generally catered for away from home. Children will often have their food provided at school or playgroup. With respect to evening meals, don't feel that you need to make a different meal for yourself while your family continues to have their usual fare. That approach demands extra time in the kitchen and reduces the enjoyment and sense of sharing that comes from eating together. At the back of this book you will find a superb collection of recipes by Antoinette Savill, which everyone will enjoy. And these menus are great for entertaining as well. There are lots of really simple wheat-free meals that you can prepare for the whole family, including young children. If you make sandwiches or other foods that contain wheat for your children and/or partner make sure that you don't sample them at the same time. It is a good idea to have some carrot sticks or a small bunch of grapes handy to nibble on instead. Also avoid picking at the children's leftovers. This is a common way of inadvertently consuming excess food, some of which may contain wheat.

Eating Out

As about one in five meals are eaten away from home these days, it is important to be aware of which restaurant foods contain wheat. You certainly shouldn't have to feel restricted when you go out to eat while following a wheat-free diet. Nearly every type of cuisine offers a wide selection of wheat-free items, so your social life doesn't need to stop just because you are avoiding wheat!

Chinese, Thai, Singapore, Malaysian, Indonesian The cuisine of these countries is on the whole wheat-free. The main staple is rice, which is served with most dishes. Noodles are often made from rice as well (such as *pad thai*). Thai restaurants are a particularly good choice, as the food generally contains lots of vegetables and very little fat. The other cuisines in this category also offer plenty of healthy meals, but some of the dishes contain fatty meats, such as duck, which are best avoided. Chinese pancakes (like those served with Peking Duck) contain wheat. As mentioned earlier, soy sauce contains trace amounts of wheat. Monosodium glutamate (MSG), a flavour enhancer used in Chinese cooking, is something to steer clear of (even though it doesn't contain wheat). Ask for your meal to be prepared without it.

Japanese, Korean Much Japanese and Korean food is wheat free, so you will have more than enough choice from these menus. Miso soup is worth trying as it is made from fermented soya beans, which have many health promoting benefits. In Japanese restaurants the thick *udon noodles* are made from wheat so should be avoided, while the thinner *soba* *noodles* are made from buckwheat, so are okay. Tempura batter is usually made from wheat flour, but sometimes rice flour is used. Unless you are certain that it contains no wheat, it is probably best to choose something else. Soy sauce is often served with sushi and sashimi.

Lebanese, North African Lebanese restaurants are well worth a visit because there are plenty of wheat-free foods to choose from and the food is basically very healthy. Most of the meze dishes are wheat free. Falafel should not contain wheat, but you might like to check to make sure. Tabbouleh is a delicious salad made from parsley, mint, tomato, garlic, lemon juice and olive oil. It is usually off-limits, as it classically contains bulgar wheat, but if they are going to prepare it from scratch you can ask them to leave it out. Pitta bread is made from wheat, so is a no-no but most of the main meals are built around vegetables and legumes, and served with rice which are just what we need as part of our weight-loss plan. Many of the meze dishes are good sources of essential fatty acids as well. North African/Moroccan food is similar to Lebanese, but it tends to contain more meat (and hence more saturated fat). Couscous is wheat.

Greek Greek food is heavily influenced by Middle Eastern cuisine, so you will find similar dishes cropping up on the menu. There are plenty of wheat-free dishes to choose from, but Greek cuisine does have a tendency to use rather a lot of oil in cooking. This should be kept in mind.

Italian A proper Italian restaurant (as opposed to a pasta bar) will have an ample selection of suitable dishes. Antipasto dishes are mostly wheat-free, so these pose no problems. Or you could have a mixed salad as a starter. Fish, seafood or meat dishes, served with vegetables are options for your main meal. Have rice or potatoes as well if you are feeling particularly hungry. Avoid bread, breadsticks and anything that is cooked in breadcrumbs. The (non-pasta) vegetarian options may contain wheat, so, if in doubt, ask. If you can't find a suitable vegetarian meal, ask for a plate of grilled (broiled) vegetables with some rice or a baked potato. Most restaurants will be happy to supply this, even if it is not on the menu.

Pasta bars pose a bit more of a problem because there is often very little else on the menu. If there is a decent salad bar you should find enough for a filling meal, but salads from the menu are usually very limited. Check out the menu in advance or you may leave there feeling hungry.

French Your options here are very similar to those on offer at an Italian restaurant. Grilled (broiled) fish, chicken or meat (without sauce) plus vegetables, salads, potatoes and rice are your main choices. All sauces are suspect as they will probably have been thickened with wheat flour. Ask for your meal to be cooked without a sauce. French sauces are usually made with large quantities of butter, so you will be saving calories and avoiding saturated fat by having your meal without them.

Mexican You will find a reasonable number of wheat-free choices at a Mexican restaurant. Corn meal is used to make tortillas and tacos in southern Mexico, but wheat flour is preferred in the north. Tacos are usually corn, but before ordering either, it is best to check. Nachos (also usually corn) with salsa or guacamole make a good starter or a light meal when served with salad. Many Mexican recipes contain rice and/or legumes so any of these are worth trying. However, Mexican dishes that contain a lot of cheese are best avoided, in view of the saturated fat content.

Indian The main food to avoid in Indian restaurants are the breads (chappatis, naan, roti) as these are made from wheat flour. Bhajees and pakoras are made from gram flour (made from chickpeas) so these are okay. Indian cuisine is generally quite healthy, as it uses a lot of vegetables, rice and dal. The only drawback is that some Indian restaurants use a large amount of oil. Tandoori meals are generally a good choice, as they are prepared without added oil.

Cafes, sandwich bars, pizza restaurants Places that serve light meals such as slices of quiche, pasties, pizza and sandwiches are going to

A FEW WORDS ABOUT RICE

Unfortunately, most restaurants still serve white rice rather than brown. White rice is fast-releasing and is not as high in nutrients as brown. However, by eating rice with slower-releasing foods (chana dal in an Indian restaurant, hummus in a Lebanese one, for instance, etc.,) we can prevent it from having a negative impact on blood sugar levels.

be difficult, as all of these foods contain wheat. It is best to avoid these venues if you can. The limited choice that is available usually consists of baked potatoes with various toppings.

Dinner Parties

Dinner parties at your home should pose no difficulties as this book offers you a wonderful selection of tasty wheat-free recipes. Most of the time your guests won't even realise that they have been served a meal without wheat. When someone else is doing the cooking, the situation can be slightly more tricky. Lots of people are avoiding specific foods these days, whether as a result of food intolerance or for other reasons, so your situation is not that unusual. When you are asked out to dinner, it is probably best to contact your hosts ahead of time to discuss your dietary needs with them. That way you can avoid the awkward situation of turning up and finding there is not a lot for you to eat. This could cause embarrassment to you, your hosts and the other guests.

Holidays

It's worth taking a few wheat-free supplies with you when you go on holiday. Useful items include a bag of nuts and seeds and some wheat-free breakfast cereals. If space permits, you could also pack some other snack foods and crispbreads. If you are self-catering and enjoy cooking, take some wheat-free flour to make your own bread. It can be difficult trying to find out whether a restaurant meal contains wheat if you are communicating in a language other than your own, so it is best to choose foods that you are sure are okay.

chapter 10

Putting it into Practice

This chapter gives you some pointers for putting this eating and lifestyle plan into practice. This is not a rigid routine that needs to be followed slavishly. There is no need to count calories or add up fat units. Instead, you have a certain degree of flexibility and can vary your choice of food according to your personal preferences. The criteria for choosing which foods to eat are based on the fundamental principles of maintaining a stable blood sugar balance, supporting your metabolism, keeping your body alkaline and making sure your digestive system and other elimination channels are clear and healthy. When you choose foods according to these five principles, weight loss should happen easily and without a big effort on your part. This weight-loss plan is based on three healthy meals a day with one or two snacks in between, so you need never feel hungry.

The foods you are encouraged to eat are both tasty and nutritious, so mealtimes will be a pleasure. We have provided you with a four-week menu plan to help you to put this programme into practice. The delicious recipes can be mixed and matched to give you an ample selection of different meals. Use the kick start plan for the first week to help you to get into the programme.

Choose Nutritious Food

Rather than choosing foods based on calories or fat units, (which can be both time consuming and restrictive, not to mention ineffective), there is a very simple question you can ask yourself that will always give a clear yes or no. 'Is this a nutritious food that meets the five fundamental principles I need to consider in order to lose weight?' If the food is highly processed and refined, loaded with chemicals, high in saturated fat, hydrogenated fat, refined sugar or salt then the answer is no. If the food is fresh and in a natural state then the answer is yes. Foods that meet these criteria will also support your overall health and well-being. They will contain ample amounts of nutrients so that you meet your daily requirements for vitamins and minerals. Just ask yourself this question before you decide to eat a particular food and you won't go far wrong.

Calorific values are misleading because calories from different foods have different effects on the body, depending on which form they come in. Foods that contain the essential fats can be relatively high in calories, but are extremely important as part of your weight-loss plan because they support the metabolism.

Get the Balance Right

Aim to make fresh vegetables and fruits a large part of your daily diet. These help to keep the body alkaline, provide a high level of valuable nutrients and are a good source of soluble fibre. Have three to four servings of complex carbohydrates every day for blood sugar support, fibre and the nutrients needed for metabolism. Two to three servings of good-quality protein a day is all that you need. Choose fish and vegetarian sources (cottage cheese, yogurt, soya, eggs, Quinoa) rather than meat, to avoid the saturated fat. Have one or two servings of essential fats per day. This equates to a tablespoon of flax seeds (linseeds) with breakfast, a tablespoon of oil on salad and a handful of seeds, plus as much oily fish (which also counts as a portion of protein) as you like.

Manage Any Cravings

A blood sugar balancing diet will significantly reduce the likelihood of any cravings, but you should also take advantage of the way in which mood foods influence brain chemicals to diminish your desire for carbohydrates. If you have a small portion of avocado, bean salad, seeds, hummus or cottage cheese about half an hour before a main meal, you will have less physical need of refined carbohydrates.

Eat Nuts and Seeds Daily

Add a tablespoon of flax seeds (linseeds) or the oil to muesli or mix with a little live yogurt. Remember to either soak the seeds overnight or grind them in a coffee grinder. Pumpkin, sunflower and sesame seeds can be added to food or mixed with almonds and brazils and eaten as a snack between meals. These provide a range of nutrients that are important if your metabolic system is to function optimally.

Proteins and Carbohydrates

For larger meals (lunch and dinner) avoid mixing meat sources of protein with carbohydrates such as potatoes or rice. Alternate your main meals between mainly-protein and mainly-carbohydrate so that you get your daily intake of both of these food groups.

Fruit

Avoid eating fresh fruit after a large meal, especially if it contained meat, as this disrupts the digestive process. Wait for at least two hours. However, it is okay to eat fresh fruit just before a meal.

Water

Drink at least 1.5 litres/50fl oz/1½ quarts of plain water every day (either filtered or mineral water). This is important to help to avoid fluid retention and to keep your elimination channels functioning properly. Increasing your water intake has many other health benefits as well. Do not drink with meals (or immediately before or for an hour after), so that you do not dilute the digestive juices. Fresh fruit juices are excellent for keeping your body alkaline. They provide high levels of nutrients. They need to be drunk as soon as you make them as the nutrients are rapidly destroyed by oxygen. One glass of freshly-made vegetable juice per day is a great addition to your diet.

Make Mealtimes a Sensuous Experience

We usually associate weight loss with restriction and deprivation. Instead, turn that idea on its head and make the act of eating a thoroughly pleasurable experience. You can achieve this by taking time over your food and by creating surroundings that are relaxing and attractive. Enjoy the unique taste and texture that each type of food offers. Food plays a vital role in our overall health, so while you are eating you might like to reflect upon the wonderful way in which your body works and consider how a particular food is going to support your health. Taking time over your food will also aid your digestive system, which will be able to process the food better.

When to Eat, When Not to Eat

Let your body guide you with respect to when and how much to eat. Two signals will support you. The first is the pleasantly peckish feeling, which is the body's signal that food is required. This peckish feeling is a genuinely pleasant physical sensation. When we eat at this point we usually get a great deal of enjoyment from our food. By eating slowly and paying attention to your body you will pick up the second signal, which is the one that lets you know that your stomach is full and no more food is required. 'Pleasantly peckish' differs greatly from 'absolutely ravenous' which is a sensation that is often accompanied by feelings of nausea, light-headedness, desperate longing for food and a slump in blood sugar levels. When we are in this state we don't really enjoy eating because we are rushing the process and, as a result, may overeat and end up feeling bloated or sluggish.

Do a reality check before you eat any food. Ask yourself whether you are genuinely hungry. If the answer is no, don't eat. Do this again during the meal, between courses; you may find that you don't want anything else, as you are already full. The only time to eat when you are not physically peckish is at breakfast or when you know that food won't be available for several hours. To avoid a blood sugar slump it is wise to have a meal or a large snack at this point.

If you find that your desire for food is based on an emotional rather than a physical need, do something else that will support and alleviate these feelings. Everyone, at one time or another, reaches for food because they are feeling a bit low. The only problem with this is that if it happens regularly it will sabotage weight-loss efforts. So, instead of eating, do something else that will help you to feel better. Pick up the phone and call a friend or put on some lively music and dance around the room for five minutes. Or do what Alan did, and write down your feelings in a journal.

Mental Imagery

Work regularly with the mental image of yourself at the weight you would like to be. Spending just five minutes a day picturing yourself when you have achieved your goal can be a really powerful way of keeping yourself on track. It will help to keep you congruent and break any patterns that lead you into comfort eating. Focus on all successes, however small. Each time you congratulate yourself for progress made, you build more momentum to keep moving forward towards your goal. Similarly, don't berate yourself if you do overeat on a particular occasion. Being overly self-critical just serves to put the brakes on your momentum and makes it harder to get back on track. Be kind to yourself. No one is perfect.

Build Activity into your Day

Create as many opportunities as possible to be physically active. These can include straightforward activities such as walking or cycling to work or more structured pursuits such as a regular dance class. Try to do some form of physical exercise every day. A minimum of three sessions of aerobic exercise a week (each lasting 45 minutes) will strongly support your weight-loss efforts. But even a brisk 15-minute walk every day can bring lots of benefits. If you decide to invest in a bouncer, get into the habit of using it for a few minutes every day. Skin brushing only takes a short time and can be done daily, while treats such as a sauna or massage can be had on a regular basis. Make sure that exercise is fun as well.

Foods to Eat Regularly

In addition to nuts and seeds, which are best eaten daily, here is a list of other foods that will support your weight-loss effort. You don't have to force yourself to eat anything that you really dislike – after all, eating is supposed to be fun – but bear in mind that your taste in food can alter quite a bit if you make a shift to more alkaline foods. Keep an open mind and have fun experimenting with foods that may be new to you. You have a vast choice, so there are always alternatives if you really don't like a specific food. For example, if you can't stand fish you can still get your omega-3 fatty acids from flax seeds (linseeds) or an omega-3 supplement. Try to make these a regular part of your diet.

- oily fish (salmon, mackerel, tuna), for the essential fatty acids that support your metabolism
- avocado, banana, almonds, brazil nuts and cottage cheese, to reduce any craving for carbohydrates
- soya products such as tofu, soya yogurt or soya milk. These are excellent sources of low-fat protein (which provide additional health benefits)
- pineapple and papaya, for the digestive system
- garlic, to cleanse the digestive tract

- black cherries, blueberries, cranberries and black grapes, to heal the digestive tract (these also contain large amounts of certain antioxidant nutrients)
- live (bio) yogurt to provide friendly bacteria for the digestive tract. Yogurt is a good source of protein
- watermelon, cucumber and celery, to help eliminate excess fluid and support the kidneys
- cabbage, broccoli, carrots, asparagus, which provide multiple benefits including soluble fibre and antioxidant nutrients. They are also very good for the digestive system
- sprouted seeds, as a source of enzymes and good quality/low fat protein
- Quinoa, for a virtually fat-free source of protein
- green leafy vegetables and nuts (not peanuts), for calcium and magnesium

A Daily Routine

An example of how the eating and lifestyle guidelines can fit into an average day is given below. Feel free to adapt the schedule according to your personal needs. For example, you can have a glass of vegetable juice with lunch if you can make it fresh at this time. Exercise classes are listed as an evening activity but you may prefer to take a class at another time of the day. Rebounding and short walks are in addition to the main exercise sessions and should be done daily.

Three meals a day, plus healthy snacks, will help to keep your blood sugar stable and your metabolism functioning efficiently. However, this guideline can be modified according to the signals that you receive from your body. Apart from breakfast (which needs to be eaten within an hour and a half of getting out of bed), meals should be eaten when your body gives you a sign that it is hungry, rather than because it is lunchtime or dinnertime strictly following a routine. There is no need to force yourself to eat a large meal if you don't feel very hungry. Follow your body's lead in this respect. Eat healthy snacks between meals if you feel peckish.

A DAILY ROUTINE

Morning
- skin brushing (3–5 minutes) followed by a shower
- use rebounder for 5–15 minutes
- hot water with lemon juice and a little honey
- breakfast (with a tablespoon of flax seeds (linseeds))
- glass of freshly-prepared vegetable juice

Mid-morning
- snack of fresh fruit with a small amount of nuts and seeds
- drink at least 500ml/17fl oz/2 cups water during the morning, plus herbal teas

Lunch time
- lunch (try to include lots of raw vegetables or salad)
- brisk 15 minute walk after eating

Mid afternoon
- snack if you are feeling peckish (nuts and seeds, hummus with vegetables)
- drink a further 500ml/17fl oz/2 cups water during the afternoon

Evening
- if exercising, have a snack 30 minutes before
- at least three times a week, take some sort of exercise you enjoy (dancing, swimming, gym class)
- drink plenty of water after exercising
- dinner
- late evening – piece of fruit if you are feeling peckish

Additional
- Pamper yourself by having the occasional sauna, steam or massage. These treats are also good for you!

The Longer Term

When you reach your ideal weight, you should find that it will remain at this level permanently, as you have shifted your set point at a steady and stable pace. You should not experience any rebound effects as you have not restricted your calorie intake significantly.

This eating plan offers you a great deal more than the ability to lose surplus weight easily. Once you have experienced these benefits for yourself and become accustomed to this new way of eating you may well decide to continue to follow most of the principles that informed your weight loss. Foods that contain hydrogenated and saturated fat have no place in a healthy diet, whether we want to lose weight or not. Nor do any foods that have lots of artificial ingredients. On the other hand, fruits and vegetables, complex carbohydrates, and essential fatty acids provide lots of health benefits other than weight loss.

Whether or not you decide to reintroduce foods containing wheat into your diet is a matter of personal preference. As discussed in the previous chapter, most people do not experience problems with moderate levels of wheat in their diet once steps have been taken to overcome any intolerance problems. However, refined flour, such as that found in white bread and processed foods, does not give your body the type of nutritional value that it requires. If you do choose to eat this grain again, it makes sense to continue to avoid refined wheat products and keep your overall intake at a reasonable level.

You might want to have another go at the 'taste test' that was outlined in Chapter Six. Put a slice of plain white bread, a piece of (organic) fruit and a small portion of any food that is highly processed and has lots of chemicals on a plate in front of you. Take a mouthful of the white bread and really focus on the taste and texture. Follow this process with the other two foods. After following an alkaline diet high in fruit, vegetables and complex carbohydrates for a few weeks it is likely that your taste in food will have changed. Many people report that the foods they previously regarded as their favourites now taste quite different and no longer appeal.

I hope that you will continue to enjoy your journey into a new way of eating and that you are already experiencing the benefits in terms of successful weight loss and greater health and well-being. As I stated at the start, the body has incredible restorative powers. It is always striving to achieve perfect health and balance. All we need to do is provide the conditions for it to do this properly. Looking after your body by giving it nutritious and healthy food will allow your body to look after you.

Dawn Hamilton Ph.D.

(For quick reference, photocopy and fix to the refrigerator, desk or diary)

Do: Drink 1.5 litres/50fl oz/1½ quarts of pure still water each day, but not during main meals.
Don't: Drink coffee, canned fizzy drinks or alcohol.

Do: Eat breakfast before work or when you get to work. Eat before the school run or when you return home.
Don't: Snack on breads, biscuits, cookies, doughnuts, pastries and chocolate.

Do: Eat salads and proteins together, or carbohydrates and vegetables together. Avoid mixing meat, chicken or fish with carbohydrates.
Don't: Add salt to your food or eat salty foods (processed or junk foods or chips/crisps).

Do: Snack on a handful of mixed seeds, nuts and raisins each day. Also snack on fresh fruit and vegetables (celery, carrots, cucumber, tomatoes).
Don't: Get so hungry that you will eat anything!

Do: Keep wheat-free emergency snacks like hummus, guacamole and smoked mackerel fillets in the refrigerator.
Don't: Eat fresh fruit until 2 hours after a meat course.

Do: Drink herb tea when you are thirsty, stressed or need warming up.
Don't: Snack within 20 minutes of a main meal.

Do: Eat salads, soups, baked potatoes or healthy dips with raw vegetables for lunch and not sandwiches.
Don't: Eat mayonnaise. Use a fat-free dressing, yogurt or fromage frais.

Do: Go for a brisk walk after lunch, but relax and unwind after dinner.
Don't: Bolt your food. Chew it and enjoy it!

Do: Eat fish at least three times a week.
Don't: Eat meat more than twice a week.

Do: Focus on things other than food.
Don't: Eat for comfort – ring a friend instead or pamper yourself in some way.

Do: Prepare food without nibbling!
Don't: Eat children's leftovers, or food from dinner parties.

Coeliacs

If you are a coeliac, you can use all the recipes in the book knowing that our nutritionist has checked every recipe. The ingredients and foods that we have used throughout the book are wheat free or with such small amounts of the starch that we feel that they can be part of our diet plan. We have indicated any ingredient that does contain or may contain gluten with an asterisk (*) symbol, so that a gluten free substitute can be purchased and used in the recipe.

chapter 11

The Nuts and Bolts

Now for all the practical information you'll need when embarking on your new eating plan. The basis of this chapter is a kick-start programme that covers a five-week period. You'll find menu suggestions for every day of the week, from breakfast to dinner, plus extra ideas for snacks, and alternative dishes for vegetarians. Recipes for all the key dishes appear in part two of the book, with variations that ensure that your diet will always be as diverse as it is delicious.

Before embarking on this new way of eating, it helps if you make a list of things to do and food to buy.

Throw out the old and bring in the new: Think of this as a wonderful opportunity to spring clean all your food cupboards, refrigerator and freezer. Throw away any out-of-date food or drink. Check every label and, if you live alone, discard any product that has wheat or wheat starch in it, so that you are not tempted to use it in an unguarded moment.

The shopping list Because most people work from Monday to Friday, the seven day kick-start menu plan begins on a Sunday, so that even the busiest person will have time to plan the week ahead, make a shopping list and shop on Saturday.

You will find quick and easy recipes for breakfast, including delicious Soda bread, Blender Shake Smoothie and Muesli. There are plenty of ideas for lunch and dinner, including vegetarian alternatives, so that you can choose what suits your budget and personal taste. The menu charts are only a guide; feel free to swap the suggested recipes around. Only you know how much time you have to shop and cook throughout the week.

Have the menu in front of you when you are making your list. Look at (for example) Sunday lunch. We suggest stuffed roast chicken but if you are on your own you might prefer a chicken breast recipe. You could make up a half quantity and have the remainder as an instant lunch next day with some salad. Alternatively, in summer, you might prefer the artichoke and chicken salad; again you can halve the quantities. Here are another couple of examples: you don't like lamb curry, so can substitute lamb chops and lots of vegetables; you don't like mackerel, so instead, have grilled (broiled) trout.

(For quick reference, photocopy and fix to the refrigerator, desk or diary)
Recipes in this book are indicated by the following symbol: ★

Week 1

	Sunday	Monday	Tuesday	Wednesday	Thursday	Friday	Saturday
BREAKFAST							
	¹/₂ grapefruit 1 thick slice rye or Soda bread ★ toasted, with maple syrup or honey	Live natural (plain) unsweetened yogurt/Yofu with 1 tsp sesame seeds & 2 tbsp berries	Boiled egg and 1 thick slice of rye or Soda bread ★	Medium bowl of unsweetened porridge/ oatmeal made with water or virtually fat-free/Soya milk with a dollop of live low-fat yogurt or Yofu	Blender shake smoothie ★	Muesli ★ with virtually fat-free or soya milk	Muesli ★ with virtually fat-free or soya milk
LUNCH							
	Apricot and Thyme Stuffed Roast Chicken Vegetables (no potatoes) *Vegetarian alternative:* ★ Butter Bean Mousse	Sandwich made with rye bread or Soda bread ★ Hummus with avocado Salad (leaves, herbs, tomatoes, cucumber etc.)	Spinach & parmesan ★ Stuffed Baked Potato ★ with mixed salad *or* Baked potato with low sugar baked beans	Mixed raw salad (anything you like) with either 100g/3¹/₂oz/¹/₂ cup tuna fish, prawns (shrimp), a small chicken breast, low-fat cottage cheese or vegetarian cheese	Three bean salad ★ and a mixed green salad	Smoked Haddock and Sweetcorn Chowder ★ *or* Fresh sardines on Toast ★	Minted Cottage Cheese with Fruit Salad ★ Mixed green salad
	★ Baked Vanilla Fruits	Fruit if desired	Fruit if desired	Fruit if desired	Fruit if desired	Fruit if desired	

	Sunday	Monday	Tuesday	Wednesday	Thursday	Friday	Saturday
DINNER							
	Cream of watercress soup ★	Leftover soup	Sliced melon	Sliced melon	Mixed salad to start if desired	Mixed salad to start if desired	
	Mixed salad with plenty of vegetables	Vegetable Lasagne ★	Seafood salad ★	Sweet pepper spaghetti ★	Tuna and Fennel Kebabs ★ (no rice)	Asparagus and Baby Broad Bean Risotto ★	Beef burger with Tomato Salsa ★
		Mixed green salad	Tomato, basil and spring onion (scallion) salad	Mixed salad with plenty of vegetables	Lots of vegetables	Lots of vegetables	Mixed salad
							Vegetarian alternative: Broccoli roulade ★
			Green salad with plenty of vegetables				Lime angel cake ★
		Fruit if desired	Fruit if desired	Fruit if desired	Fruit if desired	Fruit if desired	Fruit if desired

Week 2

	Sunday	Monday	Tuesday	Wednesday	Thursday	Friday	Saturday
BREAKFAST							
	1/2 grapefruit 1 thick slice of rye or Soda bread ★, toasted with honey or maple syrup	Natural (plain) unsweetened yogurt/Yofu & 1 tsp sesame seeds & 2 tbsp berries	Muesli ★ with virtually fat-free or soya milk	1 boiled egg with1 thick slice of rye or Soda bread ★ or Grilled tomatoes on toast	Muesli ★ with virtually fat-free or soya milk	Blender Shake Smoothie ★	Medium bowl of un-sweetened porridge or oatmeal made with water or virtually fat-free or soya milk

	Sunday	Monday	Tuesday	Wednesday	Thursday	Friday	Saturday
LUNCH							
	Salmon with roast green beans and fennel ★ (no potatoes or rice) Plenty of fresh vegetables	Sandwich with Soda bread ★ or Rye & Hummus ★ or guacamole with salad and tomatoes	Minted Cottage Cheese with Fruit Salad ★	Parsnip and Chicken Soup ★	Mixed salad of your choice with 100g/3^1/₂oz of tuna, lean meat or chicken or Hummus ★	Three Bean Salad ★	Red onion Clafoutis ★ Vegetables or Mixed salad
	★ Lemon Curd Roulade ★ with raspberries	Fruit if desired	Fruit if desired	Fruit if desired	Fruit if desired	Oat and Cinnamon Crispies ★	Fruit if desired
DINNER							
			Green salad to start if desired	Sliced melon	*Sample dinner party for 8*	Mixed salad if desired	
	Beetroot and Cumin Soup ★ Mixed salad	Lamb Curry with Spiced Spinach and Coriander Beans ★ (no rice) *Vegetarian alternative:* Wild Mushroom and Tarragon Tart ★ Plenty of vegetables	Haddock with Almond and Garlic Sauce ★ (no potatoes) Plenty of vegetables	Red Onion and Rocket Pasta ★ Mixed salad	Gazpacho ★ Broccoli Roulade and Watercress sauce ★ (make two) Selection of salads Pear and Cinnamon Slice ★ with fat-free fromage frais	Mackerel with Ratatouille ★ (no potatoes) Fresh green vegetables	Chicken Breasts Stuffed with Yellow Peppers ★ (no potatoes) *Vegetarian alternative:* ★ Quick Pesto risotto with a mixed salad Vegetables
	Fruit if desired	Fruit if desired	Fruit if desired		Fruit if desired	Fruit if desired	Fruit if desired

Week 3

	Sunday	Monday	Tuesday	Wednesday	Thursday	Friday	Saturday
BREAKFAST	Natural (plain) unsweetened yogurt/Yofu with 1 tsp sesame seeds & 2 tbsp any berries	¹/₂ grapefruit & rye or Soda bread ★, toasted, and honey or maple syrup	Muesli ★ & virtually fat-free or soya milk	Muesli ★ & virtually fat-free or soya milk	Muesli ★ & virtually fat-free or soya milk	Blender Shake Smoothie ★	¹/₂ melon filled with mixed berries
LUNCH	Roast beef and Yorkshire Puddings ★ & vegetables (no potatoes) *Vegetarian alternative:* Wild Mushroom and Tarragon Tart ★ with plenty of fresh vegetables	Mixed salad and Hummus ★ or avocado	Three Bean Salad ★	Pea and Coriander Dip with Corn Chips ★	Warm Courgette and Cumin Dip ★ & Soda bread	Fresh Sardines on Toast ★	Egg Mousse and Pepper Salad ★ Mixed Salad ★
	Baked Vanilla Fruits ★	Fruit if desired	Fruit if desired	Fruit if desired	Fruit if desired	Fruit if desired	Fruit cake ★
DINNER				Sliced melon		Mixed salad if desired	
	Sweet Potato and Ginger Soup ★ Mixed Salad ★	Tuna and Fennel Kebabs ★ (no rice) Mixed salads or fresh vegetables	Mushroom and Oregano Pancakes ★ Mixed salad	Herb omelette Fresh vegetables	Charcuterie and Pickled Vegetables *Vegetarian alternative:* Vegetable Lasagne ★ Mixed Salad	Perfect Pizza ★ Mixed Salad	Tiger Prawns with Lime and Ginger ★ (no rice) Stir-fried vegetables
	Fruit if desired	Fruit if desired	Fruit if desired		Fruit if desired	Fruit if desired	

Week 4

	Sunday	Monday	Tuesday	Wednesday	Thursday	Friday	Saturday
BREAKFAST							
	¹/₂ grapefruit & thick slice of rye or Soda Bread ★ toasted with honey or maple syrup	Blender Shake Smoothie ★	Muesli ★ with virtually fat-free or soya milk	Boiled or poached egg with a slice of wheat-free toast	Natural (plain) un-sweetened yogurt/Yofu 1 tsp sesame seeds & 2 tbsp berries	Muesli ★ with virtually fat-free or soya milk	Muesli ★ with virtually fat-free or soya milk
LUNCH							
	Roast lamb and mint sauce (no potatoes, plenty of fresh vegetables)	Mixed salad with tuna, smoked trout fillets or Hummus ★	Three Bean Salad ★	Spinach and Parmesan Stuffed Baked Potatoes ★ *or* Baked potato with low sugar baked beans	Smoked Mackerel Pâté ★ & toast or rye crispbread *or* Fresh Sardines on Toast ★	Chilled Gazpacho ★ & rye or Soda Bread ★	Asparagus and Goat's Cheese Salad ★ and other mixed salads
	Vegetarian alternative: Red onion Clafoutis ★						
	Fresh vegetables						
	Strawberry and raspberry meringues ★	Fruit if desired	Fruit if desired	Fruit if desired	Fruit if desired	Fruit if desired	Fruit if desired

Sunday	Monday	Tuesday	Wednesday	Thursday	Friday	Saturday
DINNER						
			Sliced melon			
Your choice of soup Mixed Salad	Pasta with Capers and Anchovies ★ Mixed Salad	Turkey Fillets in Mustard and Tarragon Sauce ★ Selection of salads	Chicken Breasts with Watercress Pesto Sauce ★ (no potatoes) Plenty of vegetables *Vegetarian alternative:* Tomato and Chilli Enchiladas ★ Selection of salads	Quick Pesto Risotto ★ Mixed salad	Roast Vegetable and Lentil Salad ★ Mixed green salad	Cod with Chilli Salsa ★ (no potatoes) *Vegetarian alternative:* Courgette and Pepper Tarts ★ Vegetables
	Fruit if desired	Fruit if desired		Fruit if desired		Chocolate Amaretti Tiramisu ★

Week 5

Sunday	Monday	Tuesday	Wednesday	Thursday	Friday	Saturday
BREAKFAST						
1/2 grapefruit 1 thick slice of rye or Soda Bread ★ toasted with honey or maple syrup	Blender Shake Smoothie ★	Muesli ★ with virtually fat-free or soya milk	Boiled or poached egg with a slice of Soda Bread ★ or rye toast *or* Grilled (broiled) tomatoes on rye or Soda Bread ★ or toast	Natural (plain) un-sweetened yogurt/Yofu 1 tsp sesame seeds & 2 tbsp berries	Muesli ★ with virtually fat-free or soya milk	Raspberry Muffin ★

	Sunday	Monday	Tuesday	Wednesday	Thursday	Friday	Saturday
LUNCH							
	Salmon with Roast Green Beans and Fennel ★ (no potatoes or rice)	Sandwich made of Soda Bread ★ or rye with Hummus ★ *or*	Three Bean Salad ★ with a mixed green salad	Sweet Potato and Ginger Soup ★	Pea and Coriander Dip with Corn Chips ★	Fresh (or canned) sardines on Soda Bread ★ or rye toast	Warm Courgette and Cumin Dip ★ with Soda Bread ★ Selection of salads
	Plenty of fresh vegetables	Guacamole, salad and tomatoes					
	Lemon Curd Roulade ★ and Strawberries	Fruit if desired	Fruit if desired	Fruit if desired	Fruit if desired	Fruit if desired	Fruit if desired
DINNER							
	Your choice of soup	Sliced melon		Mixed salad	Sample dinner party for 4	Sample dinner party for 4	Sliced melon
	Mixed salad with of plenty of vegetables	Artichoke and Chicken Salad ★ Mixed Green Salad	Lamb Chops with Celeriac and Leeks ★ (no potatoes) Fresh vegetables *Vegetarian alternative:* Vegetable Lasagne ★ with mixed green salad	Haddock with with Almond and Garlic Sauce ★ (no potatoes) Plenty of vegetables	★ Tomato and Chilli Enchiladas Raw vegetable salad (peppers, cucumber, fennel, chicory (Belgian endwe) carrots and celery)	Asparagus and Baby Broad Bean Risotto ★ Wild Mushroom and Tarragon Tart ★ Selection of salads	★ Mackerel with Ratatouille (no potatoes) Plenty of green vegetables
	Fruit if desired	Fruit if desired	Fruit if desired	Fruit if desired	Lime Angel Cake ★ with kiwi fruit	Baked Vanilla Fruits ★	Fruit if desired

Making the Programme Work for You

Breakfast

- Always serve soda bread toast very hot, and the bread fresh, so that you can avoid using any butter or margarine.

Lunch and Dinner

- Balance your menu carefully so that you have, for example, a very light starter before a meat or chicken dish.
- Always serve lots of vegetables so that no one notices that there are no potatoes, rice or pasta.
- End the meal with a light pudding.
- If you are entertaining but don't want to try one of the recipes in this book, serve a big mixed salad tossed in a little French dressing as a starter. You could jazz it up with asparagus or artichoke hearts. Follow this with roast chicken or grilled (broiled) salmon and vegetables and end the meal with a pure fruit sorbet.
- Make up a batch of French dressing and keep it in a sealed container in a cool place, but not the refrigerator: mix 2 tsp of mild mustard with 2 tbsp of wine vinegar and 4 tbsp of olive oil. Season with salt, pepper and crushed garlic. Use very little and toss the salad in the dressing in a bowl for maximum taste and coverage.

During the first five weeks on the eating plan, you may find it helpful to follow it closely, without making too many substitutions. On frantic days, however, when you need a particularly speedy alternative to the suggested dish, rice and non-wheat pasta dishes or stir-fries take only a few moments to prepare. Alternatively, an omelette, grilled (broiled) fish, prawn (shrimp) salad or a small steak with salad are quick and easy to make. For emergencies I sometimes treat myself to Dietary Specialties frozen pizza or pasta meals (see mail order list).

Snacks

Here are some ideas for healthy snacks that can be enjoyed between meals if you are peckish:

- a piece of fresh fruit
- a bowl of fresh fruit salad
- Rye Crispbread * with cottage cheese and cucumber
- raw vegetables, such as carrots, celery and cucumber with hummus
- raw vegetables, such as carrots, celery or cucumber with guacamole
- a small tub of live natural (plain) yogurt or Yofu
- a small handful of nuts, seeds and raisins
- Smoked Mackerel Pâté on an oatcake*
- Blender Shake Smoothie*
- muesli*

Ingredients

The ingredients used in this book are available from major supermarkets and health food stores. For those who live in the middle of the countryside, where it may be a little more difficult to find some of these products, we have provided a useful list of companies that have mail order and Internet delivery services.

The flour that was used in all the recipes is gluten free and is available from Wellfoods Ltd. This can be bought from most good health foods shops and by mail order, but at the time of writing is not available in America.

Consult the index to locate recipes when writing out your shopping list based on the 7-Day Kick-Start Plan on pages 122–8. If there is an asterisk (★) beside a dish the recipe is listed in the index. If there is no asterisk, for instance when a mixed salad is suggested, simply use suitable quantities of your favourite ingredients.

For emergencies, it is a good idea to buy extra supplies of wheat/gluten free bread, which can be sliced, wrapped individually in cling film (plastic wrap) and frozen. Then there is no need to panic if you can only manage a sandwich for lunch – but do make sure that you keep ready-made hummus or guacamole, salad leaves and tomatoes in the refrigerator for your emergency sandwich filling! You can, of course, use the recipe provided and make your own Soda Bread. It will keep for days, so you could have it for breakfast on Sunday, Monday's sandwiches and Tuesday's toast, then avoid having any more bread for the rest of the week!

Essential Supplies

Many types of gluten- or wheat-free flour for these recipes were tested for the recipes. The very best results came from Wellfoods gluten-free flour, which produces a light texture and a good colour that are less usual with most other brands. However, all the recipes can be made easily with any brand of made-up gluten/wheat-free flour.

Here is a helpful list of the most useful foods to keep in your store cupboard, refrigerator or freezer. Buy organic produce whenever possible. It is often best to buy flour, grains, seeds and nuts from health food shops, because they are fresher.

- Gluten-free and Wheat-free flour such as Wellfoods or Doves Farm (The Stamp Collection wheat free flour is available in the U.S.)
- Gram flour (from an Indian shop, use to make bhajis, etc.)
- Wheat-free baking powder and bicarbonate of soda (baking soda)
- Wheat/gluten free sliced bread
- Wheat-free ratafias (macaroons) sugar-free oatcakes*
- Rye crispbread (wheat free), Corn chips (wheat/gluten free)
- Falafel mix
- Wheat-free/gluten free spaghetti
- Rice noodles (available from Chinese or South-East Asian shops)
- Organic rolled oats*, buckwheat flakes, barley*, millet, rye flakes*, oat bran*, Quinoa flakes
- Brown or wild rice and rice cakes
- Quinoa and tofu (bean curd)
- Brazil nuts, whole almonds, walnuts and hazelnuts in their skins
- Sesame, sunflower and pumpkin seeds, flax seed (linseed)
- Ready-to-eat dried apricots, peaches, raisins, cranberries, cherries
- Canned strawberries and pears in fruit juice
- Scented clear honey
- Large free-range eggs
- Organic soya milk or virtually fat-free milk, live natural (plain) yogurt or Yofu, ice cream, fromage-frais, vegetarian cheese and cottage cheese
- Frozen raspberries, strawberries and other berries
- Frozen organic vegetables, broad beans, peas and green beans

- Frozen prawns (shrimp)
- Frozen individually wrapped chicken breasts
- Good quality pesto sauce, preferably organic
- Fresh root ginger, garlic, chillies and lemons
- Mixed dried and fresh herbs and spices*
- Worcestershire sauce* and soy sauce*
- Wine vinegar, cold pressed virgin olive oil and Dijon mustard*
- Marigold vegetable bouillon (stock) powder, dried wild mushrooms
- Canned tuna, sardines, salmon and anchovies
- Canned artichoke hearts, sweetcorn kernels, chickpeas, butter beans, kidney beans and lentils
- Canned chopped tomatoes and reduced salt and sugar baked beans*
- Herb teas
- 1.5 litre/50fl oz/1½ quart bottles of still water (or buy a water purifier and make your own)

* Worcestershire sauce, Soy sauce, organic rolled oats, barley, rye, oat bran, rye crispbreads and oat cakes contain gluten. If you are a coeliac please use alternative products.

Reference list for daily and special treats food

When you start following the programme, it can be difficult to remember which foods can be enjoyed every day, and which should be restricted. A quick glance at this list will remind you.

	Daily	Special treats only
Dairy		
Cheese, low-fat cottage	✓	
Cheese, half-fat hard		✓
Crème fraiche, half-fat		✓
Eggs	✓	
Fromage frais, virtually fat free	✓	
Ice-cream, low-fat		✓
Milk; virtually fat-free or Soya	✓	
Yogurt; natural, fat free bio, soya (natural) or Yofu	✓	
Fish and seafood All types, especially;		
Cod	✓	
Haddock	✓	
Mackerel	✓	
Salmon	✓	
Sardines	✓	
Tuna	✓	
Seafood, all types	✓	
Poultry and Game		
All lean cuts with skin removed (except roast duck and goose)	✓	
Roast duck and goose, with fat and skin removed		✓
Meat		
All very lean cuts with skin removed	✓	
Bacon, rindless grilled (broiled) back		✓
Offal, all types with fat removed	✓	

	Daily	*Special treats only*
Fruit		
All fruits, except fresh dates, fresh figs, grapes, mangoes and oranges	✓	
Fresh dates, fresh figs, grapes, mangoes and oranges		✓
Vegetables		
All vegetables, including potatoes (in their skins) and sweet potatoes	✓	
Flour (wheat-free only)		
Barley *	✓	
Buckwheat	✓	
Cornflour	✓	
Gram	✓	
Maize meal	✓	
Oat *	✓	
Polenta	✓	
Rye *	✓	
Wellfoods or other wheat free flour	✓	
Grains		
Barley *	✓	
Buckwheat	✓	
Millet flakes .	✓	
Oats *	✓	
Quinoa and Quinoa flakes	✓	
Brown or wild rice, also rice flakes	✓	
Rye flakes *	✓	
Pulses All pulses, especially:		
Broad beans	✓	
Chickpeas	✓	
Kidney beans	✓	
Lentils	✓	
Nuts (moderate quantity)		
Almonds, unblanched	✓	
Brazil nuts	✓	

	Daily	Special
Hazelnuts, in their skin	✓	treats only
Macadamia nuts		✓
Pecan nuts	✓	
Pine nuts	✓	
Pistachios		✓
Walnuts	✓	

Bottles and jars

	Daily	
Cold pressed extra virgin olive oil, sunflower oil (moderate quantity)	✓	
Natural and wheat-free sauces	✓	

Seeds (moderate quantity)

	Daily	
All seeds, especially:	✓	
Flax (linseed)	✓	
Pumpkin	✓	
Sesame	✓	
Sunflower	✓	

Sprouted seeds All sprouting seeds, especially:

	Daily	
Alfalfa	✓	
Mung	✓	

Vegetarian (wheat-free products only)

	Daily	
Soya products*	✓	
Tofu (bean curd)	✓	

Miscellaneous

	Daily	
Flavourings (natural and wheat free) *	✓	
Herbs, all	✓	
Pasta (wheat/gluten free) dried or fresh	✓	
Rice noodles, dried or fresh	✓	
Spices*	✓	

* The following flour contains gluten: barley, oat and rye. The following grains contain gluten: barley, oats and rye flakes and must be avoided by coeliacs. Flavourings, sauces, spices and vegetarian products also contain gluten and must be replaced with gluten free products.

Foods to avoid

	Avoid completely	Moderate use only
Dairy		
Butter	✓	
Cream/cream products	✓	
Full-fat cheeses/cheese products	✓	
Full-fat sweetened yogurts & desserts	✓	
Full-fat ice cream & frozen desserts	✓	
Eggs		
Mayonnaise	✓	
Custard	✓	
Fried eggs and scrambled eggs	✓	
Nuts		
Cashew nuts	✓	
Peanuts	✓	
Coconut	✓	
Coconut milk (30% reduced fat)		✓
Fats		
Lard	✓	
Margarine	✓	
Nut butters (e.g. peanut butter)	✓	
All processed meats and sausages	✓	
Items containing sugar		
Alcohol		✓
Chocolate & sweets	✓	
Dried fruits		✓
Honey		✓
Jams and spreads	✓	
Maple syrup		✓
All sugar	✓	
Ready-made cakes, biscuits cookies, pastries, muffins, doughnuts, puddings and sauces	✓	

	Avoid completely	*Moderate use only*
Miscellaneous		
Salt	✓	
Crisps and chips	✓	
Orange juice	✓	
Fizzy drinks and sweetened drinks	✓	

As these foods and liquids should be completely avoided none of the above list has been indicated as containing gluten or wheat.

60 Foods that contain wheat

This list refers to standard supermarket products. Bread, for instance, means the standard loaf, not rye bread or other specialized breads. Where the item specifies 'most' or 'many' please read the ingredients label to check whether wheat has been used. It is very important to check the labels of all processed foods, as wheat is frequently added. It may be listed as starch or modified starch.

Bagels
Batter
Biscuits/Cookies (all)
Bread (all)
Bread sticks
Breakfast cereals (many)
Bulgar wheat
Cakes and Muffins (all)
Chapatti
Crispbread (most)
Croissants
Crumble mix
Cake and muffin mix
Cauliflower cheese
Chocolate bars and sweets (candy)
Cheese biscuits (crackers) and
  Twiglets
Couscous
Curry sauce and chilled/frozen
  curries
Custard powder or sauce
Doughnuts
Dumplings
Durum wheat
Danish pastries
Egg noodles
Fish cakes or fish fingers
Fish in batter or breadcrumbs

Fish pie
Frozen desserts
French bread and French toast
Gravy powder
Macaroni cheese and Lasagne
Mayonnaise (some)
Meat pies and puddings
Mexican dishes such as enchiladas,
  wheat flour tortillas and nachos
Naan bread
Onion bhajis (but wheat-free in
  most Indian restaurants)
Pancakes or crêpes
Pasta (all)
Pasta sauce (many)
Pastry
Pitta bread
Pizza crusts or bases
Pot noodles
Quiches
Sausages and sausage rolls
Seafood in breadcrumbs
Scotch eggs
Semolina
Soup (most)
Spring rolls
Sauce mix (most)
Steamed puddings

Scones and crumpets

Sliced processed ham, turkey and
  meats

Vegetables in batter
  (e.g. onion rings)

Vegetables in breadcrumbs
  (e.g. mushrooms)

Vegetarian frozen dishes (most)

Vegetarian prepared foods (most)

Waffles

Yorkshire puddings

Equipment

These items are all optional. You will still achieve success on the programme without them, but they make useful additions and will last for
years.

Skin brush
Available at all good chemists or department stores. Needs to be made
from natural bristle.

Juice extractor
To make fresh vegetable juice. Available at any large department store.

Coffee Grinder
To grind up nuts and seeds, especially flax seeds (linseeds). Available
from large department stores.

Rebounder
Available from sports shops and department stores.

Blender
To make fruit smoothies. Available from department stores.

Plastic food containers and a lunch box
For storing food or taking food to work. Available in supermarkets.

Water filter
A much cheaper option to bottled still water. Available from supermarkets and hardware stores.

The Recipes

Sixty delicious wheat-free dishes created by Antoinette Savill
to make healthy eating pure pleasure.

**Important notice to all readers who are Coeliacs
or who have a wheat allergy or intolerance.**
These recipes aim to use wheat-free ingredients but, as they are tailored
primarily to readers who are avoiding wheat in order to lose weight,
they do include some ingredients, such as Worcestershire sauce and soy
sauce, baking powder and mixed spice (pie spice) or mustard, that contain tiny amounts of starch. For most people, these ingredients are fine
in such small amounts, but they must not be used by anyone with an allergy or severe intolerance to wheat. Items which may contain gluten
are marked with an asterisk (*) in the ingredient column. Alternatives
can be found in health food shops.

Throughout this book, all solid and liquid ingredients are given in metric, imperial and US cup measures. Please use one set of measures only,
as they are not interchangeable. All recipes have been tested twice, using
metric measures and American cups. Unless otherwise stated, eggs are
assumed to be medium.

All the recipes can be made by anyone with a reasonably well-
equipped kitchen. Any unusual utensils are listed in the ingredients column.

Introduction

The delectable recipes in this section of the book will make implementing your new healthy eating plan the easiest and most enjoyable experience you could wish for. All the recipes featured on the kick-start programme are to be found within these pages, but there are many more irresistible dishes too. After completing the five-week programme, you can continue to use the menu charts. Most of the recipe introductions suggest alternative main ingredients, so the same dish can be served in several different guises, and there's no danger of becoming bored. For example, the salmon recipes on page 172 can be made with any white fish, such as cod or tuna, or even with an oily fish. The Blender Shake Smoothie can feature any fruits you choose to suit the season, your budget and your mood.

All the recipes are wheat free. If you run out of wheat-free flour, don't be tempted to substitute wheat flour. Make sure you always have a good supply in the pantry by regularly visiting your favourite health food shop, or ordering from a mail order company. You'll find a comprehensive list of suppliers at the back of the book. It is particular important to plan ahead for special occasions and entertaining.

The recipes can be made dairy free by substituting the virtually fat-free or low-fat milk yogurt, cream and cheese products with soya products.

Combining vegetarian dishes with the fish, meat and poultry choices is a good way of keeping costs down, and you'll soon recoup any extra expense involved in buying more fresh fruit, vegetables, nuts and seeds by ceasing to snack on sweets (candies), chocolates and pastries. Use organic produce and products and free-range (farm fresh) eggs where possible.

Once you've tried the recipes once or twice, you'll discover how easy it is to halve or double them, so that your favourite dish can be served for a quiet dinner for two or a big family celebration. The only exceptions are the roulades, cakes and puddings, when it would be wiser to make two separate dishes.

Breakfast Treats

Blender Shake Smoothie Serves 1

A meal on the run! This provides an instant energy fix in the morning or an afternoon snack if you have had a very light lunch. You can change the shake to suit you or the season by replacing the berries with other fruits such as peaches and pears or apples and apricots.

- 170g/6oz/1 cup prepared fresh mixed berries (any soft red/black fruits) or about 200g/7oz/generous 1 cup of thawed frozen mixed berries
- 250ml/8fl oz/1 cup chilled low-fat natural (plain) live yogurt
- 200ml/7fl oz/generous ¾ cup chilled virtually fat-free milk, soya milk or water

- Put all the ingredients into a blender or food processor and whizz briefly. Use a rubber spatula to scrape down the sides of the bowl, then whizz again. Serve immediately in a tall glass.

Muesli

This recipe is for a very large quantity so that all the family can enjoy eating it as well. The muesli should be kept in an airtight container in a cool place. I suggest you halve the quantities if you are on your own or it may take you months to eat it, by which time some of the nutritional benefits will have been lost.

To vary the muesli, use different types of dried fruit and nuts, but keep the seeds the same. (If you have a sweet tooth, double up on the raisins.)

- 750g/1lb 11oz/6½ cups whole rolled oats*
- 500g/1lb/4½ cups combined barley*, buckwheat and millet flakes
- 200g/7oz/1½ cups whole shelled Brazil nuts, roughly chopped
- 100g/3½oz/scant 1 cup sesame seeds
- 100g/3½oz/scant 1 cup sunflower seeds
- 100g/3½oz/scant 1 cup pumpkin seeds
- 255g/9oz/2 cups ready-to-eat dried peaches or other dried fruit, roughly chopped
- 200g/7oz/1½ cups raisins
- 2 heaped tsp of mixed spice* (pie spice)
- 2 heaped tsp of ground cinnamon
- chilled soya milk or virtually fat-free milk to serve

   * These ingredients contain gluten, coeliacs please substitute with gluten free products.

- Put all the dry ingredients in a huge bowl and mix them together with your hands or with a wooden spoon. Tip into an airtight container and store in a cool place. When serving, scoop the muesli into a bowl and pour over chilled milk.
- If you leave the muesli to soak in the milk for 2–3 minutes, it will be even more delicious.

Soda Bread Makes one large loaf to serve 10,
or halve the quantities to serve 4

Low-fat yogurt replaces the traditional buttermilk in this recipe. For a savoury version, add 1 tablespoon finely chopped rosemary or grated reduced-fat hard cheese, or both. You can double the ingredients and make two loaves if you are entertaining at home.

- 455g/1lb/4 cups of wheat-free flour*
- ½ tsp of salt
- 6 heaped tsp of wheat-free baking powder*
- 4 heaped tbsp of low-fat natural (plain) live yogurt
- about 300ml/10fl oz/1¼ cups of tepid water
- non-stick baking sheet

  * These ingredients should be gluten free for coeliacs.

- Preheat the oven to 200°C/400°F/Gas mark 6.
- Sift the flour into a large bowl. Using a fork, mix in the salt and baking powder, then the yogurt. Add enough water to form a malleable dough. The precise quantity will depend on the type of flour used, so start by adding half the water and add the rest as needed. Bring the mixture together and shape it with floured hands.
- Sprinkle the dough with enough flour to enable you to knead it in the bowl to an oval or round loaf shape. If it is firm enough, this can be done on a floured board and kneaded just enough to make the dough into a smooth ball. Put the dough onto the baking sheet and cut a cross in the top with a sharp knife. Brush the top lightly with a little water.
- Bake in the centre of the oven for 45 minutes, until firm and golden on top.
- To prevent the bread from hardening further leave it to cool on the baking sheet.
- When the bread is cold, slice it and serve.
- This bread is best eaten fresh within 24 hours, but is fine for toasting thereafter. Wrap the loaves in cling-film (plastic) and they will keep for 5 days.

Raspberry Muffins Serves 10–12

These fresh and colourful muffins are perfect for breakfast. Serve them with a large fresh fruit salad and they make a quick and easy lunch.

- 285g/10oz/2½ cups of wheat-free flour*
- 1 tbsp wheat-free baking powder*
- 115g/4oz/½ cup caster (super-fine) sugar
- 1 large egg
- 250ml/8fl oz/1 cup low-fat natural (plain) live yogurt
- 4 tbsp sunflower oil
- 170g/6oz/1½ cups of fresh or lightly thawed frozen raspberries
- 12 paper cases
- 12 cup muffin tin

  *Coeliacs please use gluten free ingredients.

- Preheat the oven to 200°C/400°F/Gas mark 6. Arrange the paper cases in the muffin tin.
- Sift the flour and baking powder into a mixing bowl and stir in the sugar. Make a well in the centre of the mixture. Mix the egg, yogurt and oil in a separate bowl, then quickly pour and stir it into the flour mixture. Stir lightly until just combined. Do not over-mix or the muffins will be heavy. Lightly fold in the raspberries with a metal spoon. Spoon the mixture into the paper cases.
- Bake the muffins for about 20 minutes until they have risen and are golden brown and firm. Transfer them to a wire rack and serve warm or cold. The muffins are best eaten fresh, on the day they were baked, but can be kept in an airtight container in the refrigerator for a few days.

Soups, Starters
& Snacks

Beetroot and Cumin Soup Serves 4

This is a lovely cheerful and colourful winter soup. It freezes well, so make double the quantity, if you like.

- 1 tbsp of olive oil
- 1 onion, trimmed, peeled and chopped
- 1 mild or medium fresh hot red chilli, trimmed, deseeded and sliced
- 1 heaped tsp of ground cumin
- 3 tsp vegetable stock (bouillon) powder or 1 tbsp dissolved in 1 litre/35fl oz/ 1 quart boiling water
- 8 small cooked and peeled beetroots (beets), peeled
- salt and freshly ground black pepper
- 1½ tbsp of virtually fat free fromage frais and 1 tbsp chopped fresh coriander leaves (cilantro), to garnish

- Heat the oil in a saucepan and add the onions, chilli and cumin. Cook over moderate heat until nearly soft, but do not allow to brown. Add the vegetable stock, prepared beetroot (beets) and some black pepper and cook for about 25 minutes.
- Let the soup cool slightly, then purée it in a blender or food processor. Return it to the clean saucepan. Reheat gently, taste and add salt and pepper if needed.
- Serve the soup in warm bowls. Garnish each portion with a blob of fromage frais in the centre and a sprinkling of coriander (cilantro) leaves.

Gazpacho Serves 6–8

The great thing about this soup is that you can make it hours before serving, so it is ideal if you are rushing home after work and expecting friends for dinner.

- 3 medium cucumbers, peeled, seeded and roughly chopped
- 1 large red pepper, trimmed, halved, pith and seeds removed and chopped roughly
- 1 medium bunch salad onions or spring onions (scallions), trimmed and sliced
- 2 medium sticks of celery, washed, trimmed and sliced
- 1 small fresh chilli, trimmed, deseeded and chopped
- 1 clove garlic, trimmed and chopped
- 1 x 400g/14oz/can of chopped tomatoes
- 75ml/2½fl oz/5 tbsp fat-free French dressing
- 250ml/8fl oz/1 cup vegetable (bouillon) stock
- 2 tbsp of cider vinegar
- Extra chilli sauce if needed
- a handful of fresh basil leaves, shredded
- Tabasco sauce for serving, optional

- Process the ingredients (except the basil and extra chilli sauce) in a blender or food processor, in batches if necessary, until very finely chopped but not puréed. Scrape the mixture into a large bowl, cover and chill for at least 4 hours, preferably overnight.
- Taste the soup just before you serve it as chilling will have dulled the chilli flavour slightly. Add a dash of chilli sauce if you like, then serve the gazpacho in chilled bowls, garnished with basil leaves.

Cream of Watercress Soup Serves 4

Packed with iron, watercress has a lovely, strong, peppery taste and is perfect for soups, salads and sauces. This soup is also delicious made with fresh spinach leaves and fresh rocket (arugula) leaves.

- 1 tbsp of olive oil
- 1 large onion, trimmed, peeled and very finely chopped
- 225g/8oz/8 cups prepared watercress
- 1.5 litres/50fl oz/1½ quarts vegetable stock (bouillon) or 1 tbsp vegetable stock (bouillon) powder dissolved in 1.5 litres/50fl oz/1½ quarts boiling water
- a pinch of mixed herbs
- salt and freshly ground black pepper
- freshly grated nutmeg
- 1 tbsp cornflour (cornstarch) dissolved in 2 tbsp cold water
- 4 tsp of virtually fat-free fromage frais to serve, optional

- Heat the olive oil in a saucepan. Add the onion and cook gently until softened but not browned. Add the watercress to the pan, pour in the stock and the herbs. Bring to the boil and cook over moderately high heat for about 20 minutes.
- Let the soup cool slightly, then purée it in a blender or food processor until smooth. Return the soup to the pan and adjust the seasoning to taste with the salt, pepper and nutmeg. Bring to the boil, and then stir in the dissolved cornflour (corn starch). Cook for about 30 seconds, stirring constantly until the soup thickens slightly. Check the seasoning again and serve in warm bowls. Add a dollop of fromage frais to the centre of each bowl, if you like.

Parsnip and Chicken Soup Serves 4

This soup is a real winter warmer. On extra cold days you can always add a little curry powder or paste.

- 3 thin slices of rindless smoked back bacon
- 1 tbsp of olive oil
- 4 medium parsnips, peeled, trimmed and chopped
- 1 medium onion, peeled, trimmed and chopped
- 1 heaped tbsp of cornflour (cornstarch) dissolved in 1 tbsp of cold water
- 1 litre/35fl oz/1 quart vegetable stock (bouillon) or 2 tsp vegetable stock (bouillon) powder dissolved in 1 litre/35fl oz/1 quart boiling water
- 1 tsp chopped fresh mild red chilli
- 1 tbsp of mild, grainy mustard*
- 2 large skinless, boneless chicken breasts, trimmed of fat and chopped into bite-size pieces
- salt and freshly ground black pepper
- freshly grated nutmeg
- 2 tbsp virtually fat-free fromage frais
- 2 tbsp chopped fresh coriander (cilantro) leaves, to garnish
  * This product may contain gluten. Coeliacs please check label.

- Put the bacon in a large saucepan with the oil. Cook gently until the bacon is golden, but do not let it become crisp.
- Stir in the parsnips and onion, and cook over moderate heat for about 25 minutes or until parsnips are softened and lightly browned.
- Stir the dissolved cornflour (cornstarch) into the stock, pour it into the pan and mix well.
- Add the chilli and bring to the boil. Cook for 1 minute, stirring, then reduce the heat and simmer the soup until the parsnips are soft.
- Remove the soup from the heat, let it cool slightly, then purée it in a blender or food processor. Return it to the clean pan. If the soup is too thick, stir in a little water at a time, until it is the perfect consistency for you. Stir in the mustard and the chopped chicken and cook gently for about 15 minutes until the chicken is fully cooked and tender.
- Season with salt, pepper and nutmeg. Stir in the fromage frais and serve in warm bowls, with a scattering of coriander (cilantro) leaves.

Sweet Potato and Ginger Soup Serves 2 as a main course
or 4 as a starter

After an invigorating walk, there's nothing nicer than coming home to a
bowl of warming soup. You can make this as gingery as you like. For an
alternative you can use some curry powder instead of ginger and sprinkle the soup with a little fresh coriander, (cilantro) on serving.

- 1 tbsp olive oil
- 1 large onion, peeled, trimmed and chopped
- 2.5 cm/1 in piece of fresh root ginger
- 3 large sweet potatoes, peeled and trimmed
- 1 litre/35fl oz/1 quart vegetable stock (bouillon) or 1 tbsp vegetable stock
  (bouillon) powder dissolved in 1 litre/35fl oz/1 quart boiling water
- 250ml/8fl oz/1 cup virtually fat-free milk
- salt and freshly ground black pepper
- 1 tbsp chopped fresh parsley, to garnish

- Heat the oil in a large saucepan, add the onions and fry over moderate heat until softened but not browned. Meanwhile, chop up the
  potatoes and grate the ginger. Add both to the onions. Pour in over
  the stock and cook gently for about 15 minutes, until the sweet potatoes are soft.
- Let the soup cool slightly, then purée it in a blender or food processor
  until smooth. If the soup is too thick to blend, add a little water.
- Return the soup to the pan, stir in the milk and reheat. Season with
  salt and pepper, then serve in warm bowls. Garnish each portion with
  a sprinkling of parsley.

Smoked Haddock and Sweetcorn Chowder Serves 2–4

This is an ideal 'soup as a main meal' recipe. Serve it with the fresh Soda Bread, made using the recipe in this book, and you will have a delicious and healthy meal.

- 1 tbsp of olive oil
- 1 small onion, trimmed, peeled and chopped
- 340–370g/12–13oz fillet of smoked haddock
- 500ml/17fl oz/2 cups virtually fat-free milk
- 500ml/17fl oz/2 cups fish stock, or 2 tsp vegetable stock (bouillon) powder dissolved in 500ml/17fl oz/2 cups boiling water
- 1 bouquet garni, made by tying together 3 fresh parsley stalks, 1 fresh thyme sprig and 1 bay leaf, or 1 sachet dried bouquet garni herbs
- 2 bay leaves, if using a sachet of bouquet garni
- salt and freshly ground black pepper
- freshly grated nutmeg
- 2 x 325g/11½oz/cans sweetcorn kernels, drained
- 2 tbsp cornflour (cornstarch) dissolved in 2 tbsp dry sherry
- 1 tbsp of chopped fresh parsley, to garnish

- Heat the oil in a large saucepan. Add the onion and cook over low heat until softened but not browned.
- Meanwhile pour the milk and stock into a separate pan and add the fish, bouquet garni and bay leaves, if using. Stir in salt, pepper and nutmeg to taste. Cook over low heat for about 10 minutes until the fish is opaque and firm. Do not stir or it will break up.
- Drain the milk mixture through a sieve placed over a bowl or jug (pitcher). Discard the bouquet garni and bay leaves, if used. Put the fish on a plate, peel off and discard the skin, then flake the fish into bite-size pieces, discarding any bones.
- Add half the sweetcorn kernels to the onions. Pour in the milk in which the fish was cooked. Bring to the boil and stir in the cornflour (cornstarch) and sherry mixture. Cook for a minute or two stirring constantly until the soup thickens slightly.
- Let the soup cool slightly, then purée it in a blender or food processor. Return it to the clean saucepan. Stir the remaining sweetcorn and

the pieces of haddock. Reheat but do not boil. Taste and season with salt and pepper, if needed.
- Serve the soup piping hot, sprinkled with fresh parsley.

Note: To serve the soup the following day, let it cool and then chill it. Just before serving, reheat the soup, gently without letting it boil.

Butter Bean Mousse Serves 6

This is a delicious starter at any time of the year, or can be served as a main course in summer with lots of salads. I keep cans of butter (lima) beans in my store cupboard for salads and soups throughout the year.

- 1 x 11g/½oz/sachet gelatine (1 tbsp unflavoured gelatin) or the vegetarian equivalent, dissolved
- 300ml/10fl oz/1¼ cups of boiling hot vegetable stock (bouillon) until clear
- 3 x 410g/14½oz/cans butter (lima) beans, drained
- 500g/1lb 1oz/2 cups virtually fat-free fromage frais
- a large handful of fresh coriander (cilantro) leaves, finely chopped
- salt and freshly ground black pepper
- 2 large egg whites
- wheat-free bread and salad, to serve

- Liquidize the dissolved gelatine and bouillon (stock) with the drained butter (lima) beans until smooth. Transfer to a bowl, stir in the fromage frais and three-quarters of the chopped coriander (cilantro) leaves, and season to taste with salt and pepper.
- In a separate bowl, whisk the egg whites until stiff. Fold them gently into the bean mixture. Carefully spoon the mixture into a serving bowl, sprinkle it with the remaining coriander (cilantro) leaves, cover with clingfilm (plastic) and chill in the refrigerator until set.
- Keep the mousse chilled until just before serving it with fresh wheat-free bread or toast and salad.

Smoked Mackerel Pâté Serves 4–6

This is my favourite lunchtime snack, and also makes a marvellous nibble for serving with crudités for a drinks party.

This is also delicious made with freshly cooked or smoked salmon for a starter when entertaining at home.

- 8 small prepared and pre-packed smoked mackerel fillets, skins removed and discarded (total weight about 455g/1lb)
- juice of 1 lemon
- 500g/1lb 1oz/2 cups virtually fat-free fromage frais
- salt and freshly ground black pepper
- chilli sauce*, to taste

    * Coeliacs, please check that your brand is gluten free.

- Remove the skin from each smoked mackeral fillet, then cut the flesh into large pieces.
- Put all the ingredients into the blender or food processor in the given order and process until smooth. Scrape around the sides of the bowl and adjust the seasoning to taste and whizz again.
- Scrape the mixture into a dish. Keep it covered and cool until needed.

Hummus Serves 4

This is a perfect starter, snack or sandwich filling. You can make it as hot and spicy as you like. I alternate the herbs from parsley to fresh coriander (cilantro) or fresh basil, because I make it so often.

- 425g/15oz/can chickpeas, drained
- 20g/³⁄₄oz/scant ¹⁄₄ cup sesame seeds
- 1 fresh chilli, trimmed and deseeded and finely chopped, or a little chilli sauce
- a small handful of fresh coriander (cilantro)
- 1–2 large cloves garlic, chopped
- 1 tbsp of olive oil
- 1 tbsp of lemon juice
- 2 heaped tbsp of virtually fat-free fromage frais
- salt and freshly ground black pepper
- slices or batons of raw vegetables, to serve

- Put all the ingredients into the food processor (blender) and process until nearly smooth. Scrape down the bowl, season to taste with salt and pepper and blend briefly again.
- Transfer the hummus to a serving bowl and serve with slices or batons of raw vegetables such as carrots, celery, chicory and fennel.

Pea and Coriander Dip with Corn Chips Serves 6–8

This is the slimmer's version of Guacamole! It is ultra quick and easy and therefore ideal as a snack, starter or lunch dish. For dinner parties, serve hot Soda Bread toast with the dip.

- 255g/9oz/1½ cups frozen organic peas,
- 250g/9oz/1½ cups frozen organic baby broad (lima) beans
- 1–2 large cloves garlic, peeled and chopped
- 2 tbsp of lemon juice
- 5 tbsp of chopped coriander (cilantro) leaves
- chilli sauce* to taste or as much freshly chopped chilli as you like
- 6 tbsp of Mexican-style tomato salsa* (mild, medium or hot)
- salt and freshly ground black pepper
- wheat free corn chips,* to serve

  * Coeliacs, please make sure that these products are gluten free.

- Bring a small saucepan of water to the boil and add the peas and beans for 2–3 minutes or until just soft, cook them then drain them, rinse them under cold water and drain again.
- Put all the ingredients except the salsa into a blender or food processor and process until smooth. Scrape down the bowl and whizz again briefly.
- Transfer to a mixing bowl, stir in the salsa, then adjust the seasoning with salt and black pepper and chill until needed.
- Serve with corn chips or hot wheat-free toast.

Warm Courgette and Cumin Dip Serves 4

This heavenly concoction is perfect when spread on thinly sliced wheat free toast or with chunks of the fresh Soda Bread (page 145). Corn chips can also be used, or celery sticks if you are feeling very virtuous. As this is not suitable for chilling, make the dip within a few hours of serving.

- 2 tbsp extra virgin olive oil
- 2 large cloves garlic, peeled and crushed
- 1 medium fresh chilli, trimmed, deseeded and finely chopped
- 8 small courgettes (zucchini), trimmed and roughly sliced
- 1–1½ tsp ground cumin
- juice of ½ lemon
- 20g/¾oz/¾ cup fresh parsley, finely chopped
- salt and freshly ground black pepper
- wheat-free toast, bread or corn chips to serve

- Heat the oil in a non-stick frying pan (skillet). Add the garlic, chilli, courgettes (zucchini) and cumin and cook over moderate heat for 2–3 minutes. Shake the pan from time to time so that the courgettes (zucchini) are evenly coated with the oil and seasonings.
- Reduce the heat, cover the pan with a lid and let the courgettes (zucchini) cook until they are mushy. Check from time to time that they do not catch on the base of the pan. Transfer the mixture to a bowl and beat with a wooden spoon until pulped.
- Mix in the lemon juice and half the parsley, then taste and add salt and pepper if needed. Transfer the dip to a dish, sprinkle with the remaining parsley and serve warm with toast, bread or corn chips.
- Keep the dip covered and at room temperature if you are not eating it straight away.

Salads

Roasted Vegetable and Lentil Salad Serves 6

You can make this as a winter or a summer salad; the recipes includes suggestions for both. Vary the cooking times according to the density of the chosen vegetables, bearing in mind that winter vegetables generally take longer than summer vegetables to cook. You can double the ingredients for a party or halve them to serve 3. Use four to six different vegetables for best effect. In addition to those mentioned here, asparagus, sweet potatoes and whole field mushrooms could be used.

Winter Vegetables
- 1 butternut squash, peeled, halved, deseeded and chopped
- 2 red onions, trimmed, peeled, halved
- 2 large parsnips, trimmed, peeled and quartered lengthways
- 2 large leeks, trimmed, washed and quartered lengthways
- 2 large carrots, trimmed, washed and quartered lengthways

Summer Vegetables
- 2 small aubergines (eggplant), trimmed, quartered, sprinkled with salt and left for 30 minutes and then washed, squeezed out and dried
- 340g/12oz dwarf green beans, trimmed
- 2 large fennel bulbs, trimmed and quartered
- 2 courgettes (zucchini), trimmed and quartered
- 4 beefsteak tomatoes, stalk removed and washed

Extras
- 2 tsp herbes de Provence (mixed herbs)
- salt and freshly ground black pepper
- 2 tbsp olive oil
- 8 tbsp ready to cook Puy lentils
- 2 cloves garlic, peeled and crushed
- 1 tbsp vegetable stock (bouillon) powder
- 2 tbsp of balsamic vinegar
- 2 tbsp of chopped fresh parsley, to garnish
- a large non-stick roasting tin

Other ideas for any season are:
- Sweet potatoes, quartered
- 1 bundle of fresh asparagus, trimmed, halved
- Whole field mushrooms

The list is endless, have fun!

- Preheat the oven to 200°C/400°F/Gas mark 6
- Prepare the chosen vegetables and arrange them in the roasting tin. If you are including aubergine, sprinkle the pieces with salt and leave them to drain in a colander for 30 minutes, then rinse them thoroughly, squeeze out excess moisture and pat dry before adding to the tin. Brush or spray the vegetables with the oil, season with salt and pepper and sprinkle 1 teaspoon of the herbs evenly over the top. Bake them in the oven for about 50 minutes, until browned and tender.
- Meanwhile put the lentils in a saucepan over moderate heat and pour over with water to cover. Add garlic, the remaining herbs, black pepper and the stock (bouillon) powder. Cook, stirring occasionally to prevent them from sticking to the base of the pan for about 30 minutes, adding more liquid if needed. When the liquid has been absorbed and the lentils are soft, transfer them to a large salad bowl or dish.
- Let the roasted vegetables cool slightly, then mix them with the lentils. Drizzle the balsamic vinegar over and adjust the seasoning to taste. Serve warm or cold, garnished with the parsley.

Egg Mousse and Pepper Salad Serves 8

For a buffet or party, serve this with a delicious selection of additional salads. For other occasions, you can flavour the egg mousse with a little curry paste and change the basil leaves in the pepper salad to fresh coriander (cilantro) leaves, which will complement the flavours.

Egg Mousse

- 200ml/7fl oz/generous ¾ cup vegetable stock (bouillon) or 2 tsp vegetable stock (bouillon) powder dissolved in 200ml/7fl oz/generous ¾ cup of boiling water
- 1 x 11g/¹⁄₂oz/sachet gelatine (1 tbsp unflavoured gelatin) or the vegetarian equivalent
- 8 medium free range eggs, hard-boiled (hard-cooked), cooled and peeled
- a few drops of chilli sauce*
- 500g/1lb 1oz/2 cups virtually fat-free fromage frais
- salt and freshly ground black pepper
- anchovy essence (extract) to taste
- Worcestershire sauce* to taste
- 1 medium free-range egg white
- ½ small cucumber, peeled and thinly sliced, to garnish

    * These ingredients contain gluten. Please substitute if you are a Coeliac.

Pepper Salad

- 4 large peppers (red, orange, yellow and green) tops and bottoms removed, halved and pith and seeds removed
- olive oil
- about 36 black olives, stoned
- 1 quantity honey and mustard dressing (page 162) or ready-made fat-free French dressing
- a handful of trimmed fresh dill, finely chopped
- a large lightly oiled 2 litre/70fl oz/8 cup mould or dish, so that you can turn out the mousse onto a serving plate

- Heat the vegetable stock (bouillon) in a saucepan. Stir in the gelatine until it has dissolved completely, then pour the mixture into a jug and set it aside to cool for at least 5 minutes, stirring occasionally.
- Chop the cold hard-boiled eggs finely and put them into a big bowl. Stir in the dissolved gelatine and stock (bouillon). Add enough chilli sauce to taste, then stir in the fromage frais. Season with pepper and stir in the anchovy essence and Worcestershire sauce. Add the salt last, according to taste.
- In a separate bowl, beat the egg white until stiff, then fold in about 4 tablespoons of the egg mousse mixture. Fold this back into the bowl of egg mousse mixture. Adjust the seasoning to taste. Spoon the egg mousse into the prepared mould, cover with clingfilm (plastic) and chill in the refrigerator for 3–4 hours, until set.
- Meanwhile make the salad. Cut the peppers in half and scrape out the seeds and pith. Cut off the stems, if they are still attached. Place the peppers, hollows downwards, in a grill (broiler) pan and brush the prepared peppers with a little oil. Grill (broil) shiny side up until the skin blisters and begins to blacken. When they have cooled enough to handle, peel off the skin with a sharp knife and discard it.
- Slice the peppers into strips and put them in a bowl. Add the olives, dressing and dill. Toss well, then cover and keep the salad cool until needed.
- When you are ready to serve the set egg mousse, remove the clingfilm (plastic). Dip the base of the mould into a shallow bowl of boiling water for a couple of seconds to loosen the mousse. Use a sharp knife to ease the mousse away from the edges of the mould, then quickly turn it out on the centre of a serving dish. Decorate the top of the mousse with the cucumber, then arrange the pepper salad around the base.
- Serve immediately or keep chilled for a few hours until needed.

Artichoke and Chicken Salad Serves 4

This is an easy and delicious warm salad, which is wonderfully versatile. It tastes just as good when made with turkey, prawns (shrimp) or salmon.

- 4 large skinless, boneless chicken breasts, trimmed of any remaining fat
- 2 tbsp olive oil
- salt and freshly ground black pepper
- 1 tbsp chopped mixed fresh herbs or 2 tsp dried herbs
- 1 large clove garlic, peeled and crushed
- 8–12 frozen artichoke bottoms, total weight about 400g/14oz, thawed and quartered or 1 x 425g/15oz/can artichoke hearts, drained and halved
- ½ cucumber, peeled and sliced
- 4 ripe tomatoes, sliced
- 20g/³⁄₄oz/³⁄₄ cup watercress, spinach leaves and rocket (arugula) or lamb's lettuce (mâche), optional
- fresh coriander (cilantro), chopped

For the Honey and Mustard Dressing
- 2 heaped tsp mild mustard*
- 1 clove garlic, peeled and crushed
- salt and freshly ground black pepper
- 1 tsp clear honey
- 2 tbsp white wine vinegar
- 4 tbsp of olive oil

  * This ingredient may contain gluten. Coeliacs please check your brand.

- Make the dressing by whisking all the ingredients together in a bowl (in the given order) until smooth and glossy.
- Gently cook the chicken in a large non-stick frying pan with a little olive oil, some salt and pepper, a sprinkling of mixed herbs and crushed garlic. When the chicken is cooked through (the juices run clear when a sharp knife is inserted), remove from the heat and leave to cool.
- Put the artichoke bottoms in a saucepan of boiling water and cook over high heat for 1–2 minutes. Drain, refresh under cold water and drain again. If you are using the canned hearts do exactly the same but only cook for a minute. Transfer the artichokes to a big salad bowl and pour over all the dressing.
- Chop the chicken into generous bite-size pieces. Add to the artichokes and toss in the dressing. Mix in the cucumber and tomatoes and, lastly, the chopped coriander (cilantro). Serve warm, with fresh bread.
- For special occasions serve the Artichoke and Chicken salad on a large flat dish on a bed of watercress, baby spinach leaves, rocket (arugula) and lamb's lettuce (mâche).

Asparagus and Goat's Cheese Salad Serves 2

Home-grown asparagus is at its best in early summer, but forced asparagus is with us from all over the world, all year round, so this scrumptious salad can be made whenever it is affordable. Offer wheat-free bread when serving this as a main course.

- 1 crisp Cos (Romaine) lettuce, trimmed, washed and sliced
- 75g/2¹/₂oz/2¹/₂ cups fresh watercress, trimmed
- 225g/8oz thin and fresh asparagus, trimmed so that you just have the tender and edible top ²/₃ of the asparagus
- olive oil, for brushing asparagus
- 1 quantity Honey and Mustard Dressing (page 162) or ready-made fat-free dressing
- 75g/3oz/1 cup pine nuts, toasted until golden
- 1 x 5 cm/2 in round, ripe goat's cheese (with skin) (about 100g/3¹/₂oz), sliced in half horizontally, or a vegetarian alternative
- a pinch of herbes de Provence (dried mixed herbs)
- a handful of small, fresh basil leaves
- salt and freshly ground black pepper

- Preheat the oven to 200°C/400°F/Gas mark 6
- Trim the asparagus by either snapping or cutting them to leave only the tender top two-thirds of each stalk.
- Arrange the lettuce on two plates, with the watercress. Brush the asparagus stalks with a little oil and place them on a non-stick baking sheet. Roast in the oven for about 15 minutes or until tender.
- Spread out the pine nuts in a grill (broiler) pan and grill (broil) until golden. Tip the pine nuts into a bowl. Leave the grill (broiler) on. Season the goat's cheese with the mixed herbs.
- Arrange the hot asparagus over the salad and sprinkle over the pine nuts. Quickly grill (broil) the cheese until each piece is warm and just melting in the centre. Place a piece of cheese on each salad, then sprinkle each salad with basil leaves and a little of the dressing. Serve with salt and a little freshly ground black pepper.

Charcuterie with Pickled Vegetables Serves 6

A delicious cold platter that is perfect for parties. If you prefer fish, you could replace the meat with smoked salmon, smoked mackerel or trout, smoked eel and large prawns (shrimp). Use any fresh, baby vegetables such as baby steamed courgettes (zucchini), grilled aubergines (broiled eggplant), baby vine tomatoes and of course any pickled vegetables you fancy. Here are my favourites!

- 6 thin slices Parma ham (Prosciutto), excess fat removed
- 6 thin slices smoked lean venison or smoked, skinless duck
- 6 thin slices air-dried Bayonne ham, excess fat removed
- 6 thin slices smoked turkey, excess fat removed
- 1 small jar (about 115g/4oz) cornichons (baby pickled gherkins)
- 1 small jar (about 115g/4oz) pickled baby beetroots (beets)
- 1 small jar (about 115g/4oz) olives in brine
- 12 baby carrots, scrubbed and trimmed
- ½ cauliflower, cut into bite-sized florets
- 1 x 425g/15oz/can whole pimientos, drained and sliced or 2 large sweet red peppers, roasted and sliced
- extra virgin olive oil, preferably cold pressed, for drizzling
- freshly ground black pepper
- a large oval or round platter

- Select a huge oval or round flat dish and arrange the meats on one side of it. Drain the cornichons (gherkins) unless they are bite-size and slice them in half lengthways. Drain the beetroots (beets), cut them in half or quarters so that they are bite-size too, and drain the olives.
- Arrange the vegetables on the dish, placing them in neat rows and contrasting pickled vegetables with fresh ones: for example, start with the cornichons (gherkins), and then the carrots, the beetroots (beets), followed by the cauliflower, and finally the olives followed by the sliced peppers. Drizzle a little oil over the fresh vegetables and season them with black pepper.
- Serve with a large mixed leaf and fresh herb salad.

Minted Cottage Cheese with Fruit Salad Serves 1

You can expand this dish to feed as many people as you want. It looks great on a huge flat dish and can be accompanied by other delicious salads and wheat-free breads. When calculating how much cottage cheese to use, I generally allow about 3 tablespoons for every woman guest and 5 or 6 for every man. Aim to allow three fruits and some berries if making this for one.

- virtually fat free cottage cheese (see above for amount)
- a drizzle of runny honey
- a handful of fresh mint leaves, finely chopped
- salt and freshly ground black pepper
- fruit of your choice: such as three fruits and some berries
- 1 small ripe peach or nectarine, peeled and quartered
- ¼ small, ripe fresh pineapple, peeled and cut in wedges
- a wedge of ripe watermelon
- a handful of fresh blueberries or strawberries

   Or

- 1 small ripe pear or apple
- 1 banana, peeled and thickly sliced
- 1 kiwi fruit, peeled and sliced
- 1 ripe plum, halved
- a sprig of fresh mint, to garnish.

- Put the cottage cheese into a small bowl and stir in the honey and mint leaves, with salt and pepper to taste. Spoon the mixture into the centre of a large, flat dish.
- Arrange all the fruit around the cheese, making the most of contrasting colours and textures. Garnish with a sprig of fresh mint and serve.

Seafood Salad Serves 2

A quick and easy starter or main course, this is ideal for summer. Keep it chilled until needed and serve with other salads.

- 1 x 400g/14oz bag of frozen *fruits de mer* (seafood salad)
- 115g/4oz/4 cups fresh baby spinach leaves, lamb's lettuce (mâche) or watercress, or all three mixed together
- 20g/³/₄oz/³/₄ cup fresh coriander (cilantro), finely chopped
- grated zest and juices of 2 limes
- 1 mild, fresh, chilli, trimmed, halved, deseeded and chopped
- salt and freshly ground black pepper
- a little chopped fresh parsley, to garnish

- Thaw the seafood in a bowl at room temperature. Arrange the prepared spinach, lettuce or watercress on a serving platter.
- In a separate bowl, mix the coriander (cilantro) with the lime zest and juice, and the chilli, then season with salt and pepper. Drain and gently mix in the seafood thoroughly and fold it into the coriander (cilantro) mixture. Cover and chill until needed.
- Stir-fry the prepared seafood mixture, with all the juices, in a non-stick frying pan (skillet) over high heat. When the pan is hot, add the seafood mixture, with all the juices, and toss over the heat for a couple of minutes until the prawns (shrimp) are pink and cooked through. Transfer the seafood and juices on to the bed of mixed leaves on the serving dish. Sprinkle with parsley and serve immediately.

Three Bean Salad Serves 2

This recipe is ultra quick and easy and therefore ideal for workday lunches or manic days at home.

- 150g/5½oz/scant 1 cup drained, canned red kidney beans, rinsed under cold water
- 150g/5½oz/¾ cup canned butter (lima) beans, drained and rinsed under cold water
- 150g/5½oz/scant 2 cups fine green beans
- ½ quantity Honey and Mustard dressing (page 162) or ready-made fat-free French dressing
- salt and freshly ground black pepper
- a sprinkling of chopped fresh parsley

- Rinse the kidney beans and butter (lima) beans under cold water and drain them. Bring a saucepan of water to the boil; add the green beans and cook them for 2 minutes so that they remain crunchy. Add the kidney beans and the butter (lima) beans, to the pan and cook for 1 minute more. Drain all the beans in a colander, and rinse them with warm water and drain again.
- Put all the beans into a salad bowl and toss them in the dressing. Season to taste with salt and pepper and sprinkle with the fresh parsley.
- Serve warm or chilled, with fresh wheat-free bread or a mixed salad.

Fish and Seafood

Cod with Chilli Salsa Serves 2

Super swift recipes for nights when you get home late are a dream, especially if they are as light and healthy as they are easy to prepare. Check that the salsa is wheat free (some brands include starch). Serve the fish with a delicious green salad full of fresh herbs.

- 1 thick cod fillet, skinned, total weight about 340g/12oz
- 1 x 400g/14oz/can sweet red pimientos, drained and roughly chopped
- 6 heaped tbsp Mexican-style* tomato salsa (organic & mild, medium or hot)
- salt and freshly ground black pepper
- chilli sauce*, optional
- a handful of fresh coriander (cilantro) leaves, chopped

  * Coeliacs please check that these products are gluten free.

- Preheat the oven to 200°C/400°F/Gas mark 6.
- Check the fish and remove any stray bones. Place in an ovenproof baking dish. Put the pimientos in a blender or food processor and process them until they form a thick purée. Scrape this into a bowl, stir in the salsa and season to taste with salt and pepper. Add a little chilli sauce if you like.
- Spoon the mixture over the fish to cover it completely. Bake in the oven for about 20 minutes or until the fish is opaque and just cooked.
- Serve immediately, sprinkled with the coriander (cilantro) leaves.

Fresh Sardines on Toast Serves 2

Sardines, as we all know, are a great delicacy in Portugal. However, in Paris, my husband discovered that when a top restaurant offers sardines it may not be quite the gastronomic experience one might expect. Everyone else had ordered pâté or fois gras, but my husband chose sardines. We were all about to tuck into our heavenly starters when, with a flourish, a waiter appeared, lifted up a huge silver salver and, with great pride, presented an open can of sardines nestled against white napkins! My husband took it very well but I am afraid we dissolved into hysterical laughter, which quickly spread to the tables around us!

- 6 sardines each, depending on size, gutted, heads and tails removed, washed and dried inside and out
- coarse sea salt and freshly ground black pepper
- grated zest of 1 lemon
- a pinch of herbs de Provence (mixed herbs)
- 2 large slices Soda Bread (page 145)
- 1 tablespoon olive oil
- 1 small clove garlic, peeled and crushed
- a little chopped fresh parsley to serve

- If the fishmonger has not already done so, remove the heads and tails from the fish, wash them inside and out, and dry them well. Sprinkle the sardines with salt, lemon zest and herbs and place them on a rack in a grill (broiler) pan. Preheat the grill (broiler) to the maximum heat setting for about 5 minutes.
- Grill (broil) the sardines until the skin has blistered and become crisp and they are cooked through. Meanwhile make the toast. Mix the oil with the garlic and a little black pepper. Drizzle it over the toast as soon as it is cooked. Place the sardines diagonally across the toast, sprinkle with a little chopped parsley and serve immediately.
- Alternatively, if you are a hero, you can quickly bone and fillet the cooked sardines and lay them across the toast.

Haddock with Almond and Garlic Sauce Serves 8

I arrived home at 8pm and had 8 guests arriving at 8.30pm for dinner. The only thing that I had had time to do was buy just over a kilo of fresh haddock and a big bunch of parsley. Hence this recipe, which I whizzed up at twenty five past eight. Luckily I always have lots of frozen baby vegetables in the freezer. The instant meringue recipe on page 216 was conjured up as usual and the party was a great success.

- 1.2kg/2.6lbs/8 boneless and skinless thick fillets of fresh haddock (cod and salmon are also delicious)
- 8 tbsp of olive oil
- 4 heaped tbsp of whole almonds
- 3 large handfuls of blanched parsley
- 4 plump cloves garlic, peeled and crushed
- salt and freshly ground black pepper

- Preheat the oven to 200°C/400°F/Gas mark 6.
- Place the fish fillets in a large ovenproof baking dish, which can also be used for serving.
- Put all the remaining ingredients into a blender or food processor and whizz to a finely chopped sauce, which will coat the fish.
- Spread the mixture over the top of the fish. Bake in the oven for about 20 minutes or until the fish is cooked through and the sauce has browned slightly.
- Serve the fish in the dish, accompanied by a selection of salads or steamed vegetables.

Salmon with Roast Green Beans and Fennel Serves 2

To vary the recipe you can use any fish you like. Fresh tuna or swordfish are delicious, as are skate wings, cod, haddock or monkfish. You can also change the vegetables to other favourites such as courgettes (zucchini) or sweet peppers.

- 2 pieces of salmon (tail end fillets)
- 1 tbsp light soy sauce*
- juice of ½ lemon
- salt and freshly ground black pepper
- 1 large onion, trimmed, peeled and cut into six segments
- 2 large fennel bulbs, trimmed, tough skin removed and quartered
- olive oil
- 1 tsp mixed herbs
- 150g/5½oz/fine green beans, trimmed
- 4 medium tomatoes, any stems removed
- a handful of fresh parsley, chopped

For the dressing
- 2 heaped tsp mild mustard*
- 1 clove garlic, crushed
- 2 tsp clear honey
- salt and freshly ground black pepper
- 3 tbsp of wine vinegar
- 6 tbsp olive oil

  * Indicates products which contain gluten. Coeliacs please substitute these items with gluten free.

- Make the dressing by whisking all the ingredients together in a small bowl until thick and glossy. Use as much as you need and keep the remainder in a sealed container at room temperature.
- Preheat the oven to 200°C/400°F/Gas mark 6.
- Place the salmon fillets into a small ovenproof dish. Sprinkle with the soy sauce and lemon juice. Season with salt and pepper – cover and place in the refrigerator to absorb the flavours while you prepare and roast the vegetables.
- Put the onions and fennel in a big non-stick roasting tin. Trim the fennel and cut it into quarters. Remove any tough outer layers and add the pieces to the pan. Brush with a little olive oil, sprinkle with pepper and scatter with the mixed herbs. Roast in the oven for 25–30 minutes. The edges of the vegetables should be just blackened and the centres soft.
- Meanwhile bring a saucepan of water to the boil. Blanch the beans for 1 minute, drain in a colander and refresh under cold water. Drain again. Add the beans and the whole tomatoes to the onions and fennel in the roasting tin and drizzle with a little extra olive oil. Roast for 10 minutes more, then move the tin to the bottom shelf of the oven, so that you can roast the fish in its dish on the top shelf.
- The salmon will only take a very short time to cook (about 15 minutes), so do keep an eye on it.
- Serve the fish straight from the oven placing each fillet on a warm plate and surrounding it with roasted vegetables. Pour some of the dressing over the fish and sprinkle with the chopped parsley. The leftover dressing should be kept in a sealed container at room temperature.

Mackerel with Ratatouille Serves 2

I remember as a teenager fishing from a tiny boat off the Scottish Island of Mull and landing, to my surprise, at least 20 mackerel. As you can imagine, mackerel in oatmeal for breakfast, mackerel smoked for lunch and mackerel pâté at the start of dinner is fun for the first few days, but wears a little thin by the end of the week!

However it is tasty, very inexpensive and packed with omega-3 fatty acids.

- 2 whole mackerel, (gutted, heads removed and discarded) washed in cold water and dried
- 1 tbsp olive oil
- 1 small onion, trimmed, peeled and thinly sliced
- 400g/14oz/2 cups fresh canned or thawed frozen ratatouille
- salt and freshly ground black pepper
- a pinch of herbes de Provence (mixed herbs)
- 15g/^{1}/2oz/^{1}/2 cup chopped fresh chives

- If the fishmonger has not already done so, remove the heads from the mackerel. Wash them inside and out and dry them well.
- Heat the oil in a frying pan (skillet) and cook the onions over gentle heat for about 8 minutes until they have softened, but not browned. Stir in the ratatouille, season with pepper and simmer for about 10 minutes. Meanwhile, preheat the grill (broiler). Place the mackerel on a rack in a grill (broiler) pan and sprinkle with salt and herbs.
- Place the fish under the hot grill (broiler) and cook for about 10 minutes or until they are cooked through and the skin is crisp and blistered. Do not turn them over.
- Divide the ratatouille mixture between two hot plates, place the mackerel diagonally across each plate and sprinkle with chives.
- Serve immediately with a salad of green leaves and herbs.

Note: If you want to treble the quantities for family and friends, serve the mackerel on one large serving plate. Scatter over half the chives and serve the ratatouille in a bowl, sprinkled with the remaining chives.

Tuna and Fennel Kebabs Serves 2

Fresh tuna is so completely different from canned tuna that it is hard to believe it is the same fish. To make these kebabs, you will need wooden or metal skewers, but if you haven't got any, don't worry. Just grill (broil) the fish and fennel on a non-stick baking sheet and serve on a bed of green salad leaves and herbs.

- 2 medium fresh tuna fillets, each about 170g/6oz, skinned and boned
- 2 small fennel bulbs, trimmed of tough outer layers, both ends and then quartered
- 2 heaped tbsp English-style mint sauce
- 2 heaped tsp clear honey
- 1 tbsp olive oil
- salt and freshly ground black pepper
- 2 or 4 wooden or metal kebab skewers

- If using wooden kebab skewers, soak them in a cold water for 30 minutes to prevent them from scorching under the grill (broiler).
- Chop the tuna into neat bite-size pieces, put them in a dish. Trim the fennel bulbs and cut them in quarters. Remove any tough outer layers, then separate the remaining layers and cut them into bite-size pieces. Add them to the dish.
- In a small bowl, mix the mint sauce with the honey, oil, salt and pepper. Brush all the pieces of tuna and fennel in the dish with the mint sauce mixture, cover and place in the refrigerator for about 30 minutes, or for the rest of the day.
- Divide the fennel and tuna evenly between the skewers. Preheat on the grill (broiler) to the maximum setting. Brush the tuna and fennel with any leftover mint sauce mixture, then grill (broil) the kebabs for 5 minutes on each side. The fennel should become blackened at the edges and the tuna should be just cooked through.
- Serve immediately, with a salad or other vegetables.

Pasta with Capers and Anchovies Serves 2

You can use wheat-free pasta in any shape you like, to suit the location where you are going to eat. Macaroni or penne are easier to manage for a work lunch box, but tagliatelle is perfect for lunch in the garden with a glass of chilled Italian white wine.

- 50g/2oz/can anchovy fillets in oil, drained and soaked in a saucer of virtually fat-free milk for ½ hour to remove saltiness
- a grinding of freshly ground black pepper
- 1 clove garlic, peeled and crushed
- 2 tbsp capers*, drained (or if in salt – washed in a sieve)
- 2 tbsp good pesto sauce, preferably organic
- a little olive oil
- salt
- 250g/9oz/2¼ cups wheat-free pasta
- fresh parsley leaves, chopped
    * Coeliacs please note if there is garlic in malt vinegar.

- Drain the anchovies, put them in a saucer and pour over virtually fat-free milk to cover. Soak for 30 minutes to remove the excess salt.
- Carefully rinse the prepared anchovies under warm running water and leave them to drain. When they are dry, chop them into quarters and put them into a bowl. Add the pepper, garlic, and pesto sauce. Stir in a little olive oil, according to how strict your diet is. If the capers were packed in salt, rinse them under cold water. Drain and add to the anchovy mixture. Mix well.
- Bring a saucepan of water to the boil with a little salt. Cook the pasta according to the instructions on the packet, then drain it and tip it into a warm serving dish. Add the sauce and toss to coat. Serve immediately, sprinkled with the fresh parsley.

Tiger Prawns with Lime and Ginger Serves 4

This exotic Thai-style recipe is perfect for entertaining. You can halve the quantities if there are just two of you for dinner.

- 450g/1lb/3–4 cups of tiger or king prawns (jumbo shrimp), heads and shells removed, tails left on
- 2 tbsp soy sauce*
- 1 tbsp Worcestershire sauce*
- a dash Tabasco sauce*
- grated zest and juice of 4 limes
- 1 yellow and 1 red sweet pepper, cored, halved, trimmed, pith and seeds removed and thinly sliced
- 12 spring onions (scallions), trimmed and sliced
- 1 large clove garlic, peeled and crushed
- 5 cm/2 in piece fresh root ginger, coarsely grated
- salt and freshly ground black pepper
- 150g/5½oz/scant 1 cup baby sweet corn, halved horizontally
- 150g/5½oz/1 cup mange touts, trimmed
- 2 tbsp olive oil
- a handful fresh coriander (cilantro) leaves, to garnish

    * These ingredients contain gluten. Coeliacs please substitute them.

- Spread out the prawns (shrimp) in a single layer in a large glass or china dish. Top with all the remaining ingredients. Toss everything together, cover and marinate in the refrigerator for several hours or the rest of the day.
- Just before you are ready to eat, heat the oil in a large non-stick frying pan (skillet) or wok and add the marinated mixture. Stir-fry until everything is very hot and the prawns (shrimp) are just cooked through.
- Serve immediately sprinkled with the coriander (cilantro) leaves. If you have hungry guests or family, you could offer them steamed brown rice or rice noodles, as well.

Meat and Poultry

Beef Burger with Tomato Salsa Serves 1–4

This recipe can be adapted to serve any number of people and you can use different meats or game to suit different occasions. We frequently make venison or turkey burgers because they are so low in fat and cholesterol and have an excellent flavour. Extra lean minced (ground) organic pork or lamb is also very good. Burgers freeze well, so even if you are only cooking for one, it is worth making four and freezing the surplus separately. The salsa is enough for four but if you are only cooking for one, it is delicious the next day with cornchips or served on a salad.

For the tomato salsa
- 3 ripe tomatoes, skins removed (put tomatoes in a bowl of boiling water, scratch them with a sharp knife and then the skins will soften and come away easily)
- 1 small ripe mango, peeled
- ¼ head of celery, trimmed
- ¼ large cucumber, peeled, deseeded and finely chopped
- 130g/4½oz/¾ cup sweetcorn kernels
- 1 small clove garlic, peeled and crushed
- 15g/½oz/½ cup each of fresh parsley and coriander (cilantro) leaves, trimmed and chopped
- salt and freshly ground black pepper
- chilli sauce* to taste or freshly chopped chilli if you like hot salsa
- 3 heaped tbsp of tomato ketchup

For one burger

- 165g/6oz/³/₄ cup of extra lean minced (ground) beef (venison or turkey)
- salt and freshly ground black pepper
- Worcestershire sauce* according to desired spiciness
- ¹/₂ tsp of mixed herbs
- ¹/₂ clove garlic, peeled and crushed
- a few drops of chilli sauce* or some chilli flakes
- a little olive oil, for brushing
- (If you are making 4 burgers increase all the ingredients evenly, ensuring that you have 700g/1¹/₂lb/3 cups of minced (ground) meat.)

  * Indicates ingredients contain gluten. Coeliacs please substitute with gluten free products.

- Start by making the salsa. Put the tomatoes in a heatproof bowl and pour over boiling water to cover. Leave for 30 seconds, then drain. Nick the tomatoes with a sharp knife and the skins will come away easily. Peel the tomatoes, cut them in half and squeeze out the seeds. Chop the flesh and put it in a bowl. Peel the mango. Working over the bowl, cut the flesh off the stone so that any juice is saved. Chop the mango flesh on a plate, then add it, with any juice, to the tomatoes. Slice the celery, then chop it very finely, (ideally in a food processor) and stir it into the tomato mixture with the cucumber and the sweetcorn. Add the garlic and chopped fresh herbs. Season with salt and pepper, stir in the chilli and ketchup. Adjust the seasoning to taste and transfer the salsa to a serving bowl.
- Make the burger: Place the minced (ground) meat in a bowl. On a clean board, flatten and shape it into a circle. Sprinkle it with salt and pepper, Worcestershire sauce and mixed herbs, add the garlic and chilli sauce or flakes. With clean hands bring the mixture together into a ball and then mix thoroughly before shaping and flattening it into a burger. If making 4 burgers then divide it into 4 equal portions.
- Put the burgers on a non-stick baking sheet and brush with olive oil. Grill (broil) for a few minutes on each side or longer if you like your burgers well done. If you are using turkey or pork, the burgers must be well cooked and not at all pink.
- Serve the burgers with the salsa and a mixed salad with herbs.

Roast Beef and Yorkshire Puddings Serves 4–6

This is not only a Yorkshire favourite but a great British favourite too. Janet Woodward, who has done so much for us with the introduction of the Wellfoods gluten free flour, particularly loves Yorkshire pudding and has guided me through this traditional Yorkshire recipe.

- 1 small red onion, trimmed, peeled and sliced
- 1 tsp fresh thyme leaves
- 250ml/8fl oz/1 cup water
- 250ml/8fl oz/1 cup red wine
- 250ml/8fl oz/1 cup beef stock (bouillon) or 1 tsp vegetable stock (bouillon) powder dissolved in 250ml/8fl oz/1 cup boiling water
- 1.8kg/4lb boned roasting joint of well hung, high quality beef
- 1 tbsp mild Dijon mustard
- 2 tsp mixed herbs
- salt and freshly ground black pepper
- 1 heaped tsp tomato purée (paste)
- a good splash of dry sherry or port
- 1 tbsp of cornflour (cornstarch) dissolved in 1 tbsp of cold water
- horseradish sauce or mustard* to serve

For the Yorkshire puddings
- 110g/4oz/1 cup of wheat-free flour*, sifted
- a pinch each of salt and freshly ground black pepper
- 1 medium or large free-range egg
- 300ml/10fl oz/1¼ cups virtually fat-free milk
- very little vegetable oil for greasing
- 1 x 6 large, bun/muffin tin or 8 small tins to provide 1 or 2 puddings each according to who is dieting!

  * These ingredients may contain gluten and should be checked by all Coeliacs.

- Preheat the oven to 200°C/400°F/Gas mark 6.
- Make the Yorkshire pudding batter. Mix the flour, salt and pepper in a bowl and make a well in the centre. Break in the egg, pour in half the milk and beat with a wooden spoon, gradually incorporate in the surrounding flour, until the mixture is smooth. Gradually beat in the

remaining milk until the batter is really smooth and the surface is covered with tiny bubbles. Pour the batter into a jug (pitcher). Cover and leave in the refrigerator for at least 30 minutes.

- Meanwhile, spread out the red onion slices in a roasting tin. Sprinkle them with thyme then add the water, red wine and stock (bouillon). Spread the fat of the beef with the mustard; sprinkle it with the mixed herbs and season with salt and pepper. Place the beef on the onions, with the fat side uppermost, so that it will get brown and crisp.
- Put the beef into the oven. If you like your meat rare, roast for 50 minutes, which is 10 minutes per 455g/1lb plus 10 minutes; for well-done meat, give it $1^1/_4$ hours, which is 15 minutes per 455g/1lb. On top of this the beef will need 15 minutes resting time, when the meat will continue to cook and the flavours develop.
- The puddings will take about 15 minutes to cook, so they should go into the oven when the beef comes out. About 5 minutes before the beef is cooked, increase the oven temperature to 240°C/475°F/Gas mark 9. This will not harm the beef. Take it out of the oven at the correct time and transfer it to a heated platter. Cover with a foil tent and leave to rest while you cook the puddings. Set the roasting tin aside.
- Put a little drop of oil into each of the tins and heat them in the oven until the oil is smoking hot. Meanwhile, briefly beat the batter with a wooden spoon. As soon as the tins are hot enough, remove them from the oven and pour in the batter as quickly as you can. Put them straight into the oven and bake for 15 minutes, by which time they should be well risen, puffy and golden. If in doubt keep them in the oven for 5 minutes more.
- Meanwhile, back to the beef, take it out of the roasting tin and transfer it onto a carving plate or board.
- Now make the gravy. Drain the excess fat from the juices in the roasting tin and transfer it to the top of the stove. Over a moderate heat, stir in the tomato purée (paste), sherry or port and the prepared cornflour (cornstarch) mixture. Stir the gravy scraping in any sediment on the base of the roasting tin, until it reaches boiling point. Continue to cook for a minute or two. When the gravy is thick, adjust the seasoning and transfer it to a warm gravyboat.
- Slice the beef thinly and serve it with the Yorkshire puddings, plenty of lightly cooked vegetables and the gravy. This Sunday lunch is traditionally served with horseradish sauce or mustard.

Lamb Curry with Spiced Spinach Serves 8

Next time you fancy a curry and rice with naan bread and poppadoms, try a less fattening feast and enjoy the curry with spiced spinach, beans with crushed coriander and low-fat minted fromage frais. If you are serving very hungry guests, add steamed brown rice with fresh coriander (cilantro) leaves.

- 2 tbsp olive oil
- 3 large onions, trimmed, peeled and chopped
- 2 tbsp tandoori masala powder or similar spice mixture
- 5 kaffir lime leaves
- 2.5 cm/1 in piece fresh root ginger, coarsely grated
- 1 heaped tsp cardamom pods, cracked open
- salt and freshly ground black pepper
- 3 cloves garlic, peeled and crushed
- 2 x 400g/14oz/cans chopped tomatoes in juice
- 800g/1lb 12oz/4 cups cubed, fillet end of leg of lamb, excess fat removed

For the minted fromage frais
- 500g/1lb 1oz/2 cups virtually fat-free fromage frais
- 2–3 tbsp chopped fresh mint leaves
- 2 cloves garlic, peeled and crushed
- salt and freshly ground black pepper

For the beans with crushed coriander
- 400g/14oz dwarf green beans, trimmed
- 1 tbsp olive oil
- 1 tbsp coriander seeds, crushed

For the spiced spinach
- 1 red onion, trimmed, peeled and finely chopped
- 1 tbsp of olive oil
- 1 tbsp of cumin seeds
- 310g/11oz/5–6 cups fresh baby spinach leaves, washed
- finely grated zest and juice of 1 lime

- Make the curry first: Heat the oil in a large, heavy saucepan over moderate heat and cook the onions until softened but not browned. Stir in the masala powder, the lime leaves and the ginger. Scrape the tiny seeds out of the cardamom pods and stir them into the onions with salt, pepper and garlic. Cook over moderate heat for 2–3 minutes, then pour in the tomatoes and juice. Reduce the heat slightly, cover the saucepan with a lid and simmer for 10 minutes.
- If you are preparing this in advance, stir in the lamb and cook for 50 minutes. Cool then chill for up to 24 hours. To serve, reheat for about 50 minutes or until the meat is tender and the sauce has thickened and is very hot.
- If you are going to serve the curry straight away, cook it for about $1^1/2$ hours or until the meat is tender, and the sauce has thickened.
- While the sauce is cooking, make the minted fromage frais by combining all the ingredients in a serving bowl. Cover and chill until needed.
- Cook the beans. Heat the oil in a frying pan and toss them over moderate heat with the coriander seeds until lightly browned and just about soft. Season to taste with salt and pepper and transfer to a hot dish, Keep hot while you cook the spinach.
- Heat the oil in a big saucepan and fry the onion over moderate heat until soft. Stir in the cumin seeds, then add the spinach. The heat will wilt the spinach very quickly. As soon as it has cooked down to about half the original size, stir in the lime zest and juice and season to taste with salt and pepper. Transfer to a hot dish and serve immediately, with the curry, the beans and the minted fromage frais.

Lamb Chops with Celeriac and Leeks Serves 2–4

The joy of this recipe is that you can replace the lamb chops with pork chops (trimmed of fat), veal chops, chicken breasts (with skin) or thick salmon steaks. Adjust the timing accordingly. If you use chicken, remove the skin when eating.

- 1 tbsp olive oil, plus extra for brushing chops
- 2 whole large leeks, trimmed, sliced, washed and dried
- 1 medium celeriac, peeled and quartered
- freshly ground black pepper and freshly grated nutmeg
- 300ml/10fl oz/1¼ cups vegetable stock (bouillon) or 1 tbsp stock (bouillon) powder dissolved in 300ml/10fl oz/1¼ pints boiling water
- 2 large cloves garlic, peeled and crushed
- 2 tsp dried mixed herbs
- a sprinkling of cayenne pepper
- 4–8 lamb chops
- 30 cm/12 in oval baking dish

- Preheat oven to 200°C/400°F/Gas mark 6.
- Heat the oil and add the prepared leeks. Cook in a saucepan for 3–4 minutes over moderate heat until they have softened, but not brown.
- Meanwhile peel the celeriac and slice it thinly. Bring a pan of water to the boil and cook the celeriac for 1 minute, until just softened. Drain the celeriac, rinse under cold water, and drain again.
- Cover the base of a baking dish with half the celeriac slices. Season with pepper and nutmeg. Cover the celeriac with all the leeks and repeat the seasoning. Spread out the remaining celeriac slices on top and repeat the seasoning.
- Pour the prepared stock (bouillon) evenly over the vegetables and sprinkle with half the crushed garlic, half the herbs and all the cayenne pepper. Bake in the oven for 45 minutes, then arrange the lamb chops over the vegetables. Brush the chops with olive oil and sprinkle with the remaining garlic, herbs and some pepper.
- Return the dish to the oven and bake for a further 30 minutes. Let the dish settle for a couple of minutes before serving with plenty of green vegetables.

Tomato and Chilli Enchiladas Serves 6

At last! Mexican food you can enjoy at home! Making your own tortillas with wheat-free flour isn't difficult. This recipe produces soft flatbreads that are difficult to distinguish from the traditional Mexican variety. The filling can be made with minced (ground) beef, turkey or chicken instead of pork. For a vegetarian version, simply substitute 1 × 400g/14oz can organic, wheat-free baked beans and 1 × 400g/14oz can kidney beans (drained) for the pork. The tortillas freeze beautifully, either freshly made or layered with the filling.

- 225g/8oz/2 cups wheat-free flour*, plus extra for kneading and rolling dough
- 25g/1oz/2 tbsp lard (hard white vegetable shortening)
- 1 tsp salt
- 185ml/6fl oz/3–4 cups warm water
- 2 hearts Cos (Romaine) lettuce, shredded
- 2 ripe avocados, halved, peeled, seeded and roughly chopped
- 4 tbsp chopped fresh coriander (cilantro)
- freshly ground black pepper
- extra virgin olive oil, for drizzling
- 500g/1lb 1oz/2 cups half-fat crème fraiche

For the filling
- 1 tbsp olive oil
- 2 medium onions, trimmed, peeled and finely chopped
- 340g/12oz/1½ cups extra lean minced (ground) pork
- 1 × 400g/14oz can chopped tomatoes
- chilli flakes or powder to taste
- 2 cloves garlic, peeled and crushed
- 1–1½ tsp ground cumin
- 2 tsp dried oregano
- 1 tsp caster (superfine) sugar

For the topping
- 1 × 330ml/11fl oz/scant 1½ cups V8 vegetable juice or tomato juice
- 170g/6oz/1½ cups grated half-fat cheese or vegetarian equivalent
- cayenne pepper

   * This ingredient may contain gluten.

- Make the tortillas about $2^1/2$ hours before you plan to serve the finished dish. Sift the flour into a medium bowl and rub in the lard with your fingertips until it resembles fine breadcrumbs. Make a well in the centre of the mixture. Dissolve the salt in the warm water, then pour it into the well. Mix with your hands, gradually incorporating the surrounding flour mixture to make a soft dough. Turn this on to a floured board and knead for 2–3 minutes, then place in a floured bowl, cover with clingfilm (plastic wrap) and leave to rest for 2 hours.
- Meanwhile, make the filling. Heat the oil in a frying pan (skillet) and fry the onions until soft and translucent, but not browned. Stir in the minced (ground) pork and cook for 2–3 minutes, stirring occasionally. Mix in the tomatoes, chilli flakes or powder, garlic, cumin, oregano and sugar. Season with salt and pepper. Simmer for 20 minutes, stirring occasionally until the pork is fully cooked, then switch off the heat and leave the mixture to cool down slowly.
- Turn the dough out on to a floured surface, knead for 1 minute, then divide into 12 balls. Keep these covered under clingfilm (plastic wrap) while you make each tortilla in turn. Flour the surface again and roll out one of the balls to an 18 cm/7 in paper-thin round, giving the dough a quarter turn each time you roll it. Repeat with the remaining dough balls, covering the finished tortillas with clingfilm (plastic wrap) so that they do not dry out.
- Heat a 20 cm/8 in non-stick frying pan over medium-high heat. Add a tortilla and cook for 30–40 seconds until bubbles appear on the surface and the underside is speckled with brown. Do not overcook, or the tortilla will be too dry to roll. Slide the tortilla on to a plate and cover with a piece of baking parchment. Cook the remaining tortillas in the same way, stacking them on the plate with a piece of parchment between each. Preheat the over to 200°C/400°F/gas mark 6.
- Fill each tortilla with about 2 tablespoons of the filling and roll up. Arrange them in a single layer in a very large ovenproof serving dish. Pour the vegetable juice or tomato juice for the topping around the tortillas, then sprinkle them with the cheese. Add a dusting of cayenne. Bake for 15 minutes or until the filled tortillas are bubbling hot.
- Mix the shredded lettuce with the avocado and coriander (cilantro) in a bowl. Drizzle lightly with olive oil and season with salt and pepper.
- Serve the enchiladas with a bowl of crème fraiche and accompany them with the lettuce.

Chicken Breasts in Watercress Pesto Sauce Serves 4

If you are in a tearing hurry you can, of course, use a fresh ready-made (wheat-free) pesto sauce, but not the sort that comes in a jar and keeps for a long time, as the consistency would be wrong. You can substitute watercress for rocket (arugula), with equally delicious results.

- 4 small leeks, trimmed and sliced
- 4 chicken breasts (preferably from corn-fed birds), skinned and trimmed of fat
- 1 small fresh red chilli (medium or mild), trimmed, deseeded and sliced

For the Pesto
- 1–2 cloves garlic, peeled and quartered
- 2 large handfuls trimmed, fresh watercress
- 1 large handful fresh basil
- 1 large handful fresh parsley
- 1 large handful toasted pine nuts
- 1 large handful coarsely grated Parmesan cheese (or reduced fat hard cheese)
- olive oil
- salt and freshly ground black pepper

- Preheat the oven to 200°C/400°F/Gas mark 6
- Make the pesto sauce. Spread out the pine nuts in a grill (broiler) pan and place under moderate heat until golden, shaking the pan occasionally. Cool, then put the nuts in a food processor or blender. Add the watercress, basil and parsley. Process briefly, then, with the machine running, pour in the oil through the feeder tube until the ingredients are finely chopped and you have a spreadable sauce. Season with salt and pepper to taste.
- Spread out the leeks on the base of a baking dish that is large enough to hold the chicken breasts side by side. Add the chicken breasts, making sure that they do not touch. Spread the pesto sauce over the chicken breasts, then sprinkle them with the chilli.
- Bake the chicken in the oven for 35–40 minutes or until it is cooked through and the leeks are soft.
- Serve immediately, with salad or vegetables.

Chicken Breasts stuffed with Yellow Peppers Serves 2

This dish creates its own juices, so there is no need to make an additional sauce. To serve 4, simply double the ingredients.

- 2 large chicken breasts, preferably from corn-fed birds, skinned and trimmed of fat
- 1 large yellow pepper, top and bottom removed, halved, pith and seeds removed
- salt and freshly ground black pepper
- 1 large clove garlic, peeled and crushed
- a small bunch of fresh basil
- 4 thin slices rindless smoked back bacon, excess fat removed
- a little olive oil
- a large pinch of dried mixed herbs

- Preheat the oven to 200°C/400°F/Gas mark 6.
- Carefully slice through each chicken breast lengthways until you can open it out flat. Cut the pepper into finger-sized slices. Place a couple of these on one half of each chicken breast and season with salt and pepper. Sprinkle with the garlic and cover the pepper pieces with basil leaves. Bring the uncovered chicken piece over and mould the breast to its original shape. Wrap two slices of bacon around each breast so that it is totally covered, then drizzle or spray with a very little olive oil. Sprinkle each filled breast with mixed herbs.
- Scatter the remaining pepper sticks in a baking dish that is large enough to hold the chicken breasts side by side. Place the chicken on top.
- Bake for about 35–45 minutes, or until the bacon is crisp and the chicken and peppers are cooked through. Serve straight away, with the juices.

Apricot and Thyme stuffed Roast Chicken Serves 6–8

As we suggest you do not mix carbohydrates with protein for the biggest meal of the day, this is a vegetable, fruit and nut stuffing. You can substitute a small turkey if you prefer. Choose one that weighs 2.3–2.7kg/5–6lb.

- 1 large free-range chicken, about 2.4kb/5.3lb
- 2 tbsp olive oil, plus extra for drizzling
- 3–4 leeks, about 565g/1¼lb, finely chopped
- 250g/9oz/2 cups ready-to-eat dried apricots, finely chopped
- 115g/4oz/1 cup pecan nut pieces, finely chopped
- 2 tsp fresh or dried thyme leaves
- salt and freshly ground black pepper
- freshly grated nutmeg
- grated zest ½ a lemon
- 30g/1oz/1 cup fresh parsley
- 1 small egg, beaten
- 200ml/7fl oz/1¾ cups of white wine and 400ml/14floz/1¾ cups water or chicken stock (bouillon)
- 1 tsp vegetable stock (bouillon)
- 1 tbsp cornflour (cornstarch) dissolved in 2 tbsp of cold water

- Preheat the oven to 200°C/400°F/Gas mark 6.
- Remove any giblets or pockets of fat from inside the chicken, and discard. If there is any trussing string, remove it. Wash and dry your hands and, with the back of the chicken facing you, lift up the skin from the base and gently ease it away from the flesh.
- Use your thumbs to start with, and then your fingers, to work up to the far top point. Be careful not to tear the skin, as you will be putting the stuffing underneath it. Wash and dry your hands again.
- Heat the olive oil in a saucepan, add the leeks and cook over moderate heat for 10 minutes until just softened. Stir in the chopped apricots, pecans and thyme, season to taste with salt and pepper and nutmeg, grated lemon zest and chopped parsley. Remove the stuffing from the heat, cool for 10 minutes and then stir in the beaten egg. Leave the stuffing until it is cool enough to handle.
- With clean hands, push all the stuffing under the chicken skin, moulding and flattening it as you do so. Pull the flap of skin over and tuck it underneath the chicken, as this will help to prevent the stuffing from leaking out.
- Place the chicken into a roasting tin and pour in the white wine and water or stock (bouillon). Drizzle a little olive oil over the skin of the chicken and dust lightly with black pepper.
- Roast in the oven for about 1½ hours. Halfway through cooking you will probably need to top up the pan juices with more water or chicken stock. When the chicken is cooked, remove it from the pan and leave to stand on a carving board for 10 minutes while you make some gravy and cook the vegetables.
- In a small bowl, mix the stock (bouillon) powder with the cornflour (cornstarch) mixture. Skim off any excess fat from the juices in the roasting pan, then place it over medium heat. Add the contents of the bowl and bring to the boil, stirring constantly and scraping the bottom of the roasting tin to incorporate all the flavours from the sediment. When the gravy has thickened pour it into a gravyboat and keep hot. Carve the chicken, and serve it with the stuffing, gravy and vegetables.

Turkey Fillets in Mustard and Tarragon Sauce Serves 4

This recipe is just as easy with chicken breasts and is delicious served with steamed vegetables or a crisp mixed salad.

- 2 tbsp olive oil
- 1 tbsp fresh tarragon leaves, or 2 tsp dried tarragon leaves
- 1 small red onion, trimmed, peeled and chopped
- salt and freshly ground black pepper
- freshly grated nutmeg
- 125ml/4fl oz/½ cup dry sherry
- 250ml/8fl oz/1 cup vegetable stock (bouillon)
- 4 thick, raw turkey fillets or 8 small, trimmed of fat and skin
- 1 tbsp cornflour (cornstarch) dissolved in 2 tsp cold water
- 1 tbsp very mild Dijon mustard*
- 2–3 tbsp virtually fat-free fromage frais
- a handful of fresh parsley, trimmed and chopped

  * Mustard may contain gluten and therefore all Coeliacs should check the label.

- Heat the oil with the tarragon in a large non-stick frying pan (skillet). Add the onion and cook gently until it is nearly soft, but not brown. Season with salt, pepper and nutmeg and stir in the sherry. Cook over moderate heat for 2–3 minutes, then stir in the stock (bouillon).
- Add the turkey fillets and simmer for 15–20 minutes until they are tender and fully cooked. Lift out the turkey fillets and put them on a warm serving dish. Keep hot for a few minutes while you make the sauce.
- Increase the heat and stir the cornflour (cornstarch) mixture and water into the juices remaining in the pan. Bring to the boil. Cook the sauce until it boils and thickens, then reduce the heat and stir in the mustard and lastly the fromage frais. Season to taste and spoon the sauce over the turkey fillets.
- Sprinkle with the chopped parsley and serve immediately, accompanied by lots of steamed fresh vegetables.

Vegetable and Vegetarian Dishes

Red Onion and Rocket Pasta Serves 2

A delicious addition to this pasta dish would be steamed courgettes (zucchini) or slices of goat's cheese and fresh basil.

- 170g/6oz/2 cups wheat-free dried macaroni or pasta shapes
- 2 tbsp olive oil
- 2 red onions, trimmed, peeled and cut into 8 segments
- 1 tsp herbes de Provence (mixed herbs)
- salt and freshly ground black pepper
- 1 large clove garlic, peeled and crushed
- grated zest and juice of 1 lemon
- 2 large handfuls of fresh rocket (arugula)
- 2 handfuls of grated half fat hard cheese or vegetarian equivalent

- Cook the pasta in boiling water according to the instructions on the packet. Meanwhile, heat the oil in a saucepan and cook the onions over high heat until they are soft and have begun to brown at the edges. Stir in the herbs, season with the salt and pepper, then add the garlic, lemon zest and juice. Remove from the heat. Drain the pasta and tip it into a serving bowl. Add the onions and toss to mix, then quickly mix in the rocket (arugula). Sprinkle with the cheese and serve immediately.

Asparagus and Broad Bean Risotto Serves 2 as a main course, or 4 as a starter

If asparagus is out of season, or too expensive, try trimmed mangetouts (snow peas) or sugar snaps, or trimmed and halved fine green beans instead.

Risotto
- 24 asparagus stalks
- 1 tbsp olive oil
- 1 medium onion, peeled and trimmed and finely chopped
- 240g/8oz/1⅓ cups/4 handfuls risotto rice
- 125ml/4fl oz/½ cup white wine
- 500ml/17fl oz/2 cups vegetable stock (bouillon), or 1 tbsp vegetable stock (bouillon) powder dissolved in 500ml/17fl oz/2 cups boiling water, plus an extra 250ml/8fl oz/1 cup boiling water
- 200g/7oz/1¼ cups of baby broad beans

For the pesto sauce
- 75g/2½oz/2½ cups fresh coriander (cilantro)
- 50g/2oz/⅔ cup pine nuts
- 2 tbsp olive oil
- salt and freshly ground black pepper

- Trim the asparagus by either snapping or cutting them to leave only the tender top two-thirds of each stalk. Heat the oil in a large saucepan and cook the onions over moderate heat until softened, but not browned. Stir in the rice and cook for 30 seconds, then add the wine. Cook the mixture for about 30 seconds more, then stir in the prepared stock (bouillon). Bring to the boil and cook for 7 minutes, then reduce the heat so that the rice simmers. Cook it for 10 minutes more. When most of the liquid has evaporated, add the extra boiling water. Continue to simmer the mixture gently, stirring it from time to time to prevent it from sticking to the bottom of the pan.
- Meanwhile, bring two saucepans of water to the boil. Cut each asparagus stalk into three pieces, then cook the asparagus in one saucepan and the broad beans in the other. The vegetables should be *al dente* – just cooked through.
- While the vegetables are cooking make the pesto sauce. Put the coriander (cilantro), pine nuts and olive oil into a blender or food processor and process until smooth. Scrape around the bowl, season with salt and pepper and whizz again.
- As soon as the rice is plump and soft, fold in the broad beans, then the pesto sauce, and lastly (and very gently) the asparagus.
- Serve in a warm dish and accompany with a mixed salad.

Broccoli Roulade and Watercress Sauce Serves 8 as a starter;
4 as a main course

This makes a nice change from spinach roulade and makes a colourful vegetarian dish for a buffet.

- 400g/14oz/4 cups roughly chopped broccoli
- juice ½ lemon
- 4 large eggs, separated
- salt and freshly ground black pepper
- freshly grated nutmeg
- poppy seeds or sesame seeds, for sprinkling
- 150g/5oz/generous 1 cup drained, canned sweetcorn kernels
- 250g/9oz/scant 1 cup virtually fat-free fromage frais
- fresh herbs, to garnish

For the watercress sauce
- 100g/3½oz/4 handfuls fresh watercress leaves and stalks, washed
- finely grated rind of one lime and the juice of ½ a lime
- a pinch of sugar
- 500g/1lb 1oz/2 cups virtually fat-free fromage frais
- a 28 x 35 cm/11 x 14 in Swiss roll tin (jelly roll pan) lined with baking parchment or greaseproof (wax) paper

- Preheat the oven to 200°C/400°F/Gas mark 6.
- Make the watercress sauce first by whizzing all the ingredients together in a blender or food processor until smooth. Season with the salt and pepper, blend briefly again, then pour into a jug (pitcher), cover and chill until needed.
- Bring a saucepan of water to the boil and cook the broccoli for 3–4 minutes, until soft. Drain, cool and then purée in a blender or food processor with the lemon juice. Blend in the egg yolks, then transfer to a big bowl and season with salt, pepper and nutmeg.
- In a separate bowl, whisk the egg whites until stiff. Fold them into the purée. Lightly spread the mixture in the prepared tin. Bake for about 12 minutes or until the roulade is firm to touch and golden. Cover the roulade with a clean cloth and leave it in the tin for 5 minutes. Meanwhile cut a piece of baking parchment or greaseproof (wax) paper slightly larger than the tin. Sprinkle it with poppy seeds or sesame seeds. Remove the cloth from the roulade, then invert it onto the prepared piece of paper. Quickly peel the lining paper off the roulade. Quickly roll up this used bit of paper into a sausage and roll the roulade around it, pulling it towards you and using the seed-covered paper as a guide. Cover with a clean cloth and leave until the roulade is cold.
- Make the filling by mixing the sweetcorn and fromage frais together in a bowl. Season to taste with salt and pepper.
- Unroll the roulade and carefully remove the sausage-shaped paper. Quickly and gently spread the filling all over the roulade. Then, using the paper underneath to guide you, roll the roulade towards you until it is the shape of a Swiss (jelly) roll. Slide the roulade carefully on to a serving dish and garnish with fresh herbs. Serve the roulade in slices, with the chilled sauce. If you are serving the roulade later, mould some clingfilm (plastic wrap) around it so that it retains its shape and does not crack.

Courgette and Pepper Tarts Serves 6 as a main course, or 12 for a party

These tarts are very adaptable. I make them cold for picnics and hot for dinner parties.

- 200g/7oz/2 generous cups of wheat-free flour*, plus extra for rolling pastry
- 2 tsp mild Dijon mustard*
- salt and freshly ground black pepper
- cayenne pepper
- 100g/3½oz/generous ½ cup vegetable margarine
- 1 large egg
    * Coeliacs, please check label as these may contain gluten.

For the filling
- 1 tbsp olive oil
- 1 onion, trimmed, peeled and finely chopped
- 2 small sweet peppers, 1 yellow and 1 red, cored, seeded and chopped into the same size pieces as the onions
- 2 pinches of herbs de Provence (mixed herbs)
- 1 courgette (zucchini), trimmed and chopped to match the onions and peppers
- 1 large clove garlic, peeled and crushed
- 370g/13oz/1½ cups low-fat set Greek-style yogurt
- 2 large eggs
- cayenne pepper
- 6 x 10 cm/4 in tartlet tins or 1 x 12-cup muffin tin

- Preheat the oven to **200°C/400°F/Gas mark 6**.
- Line the tart or muffin **tins** with circles of baking parchment. Put the flour, mustard, salt, **pepper,** cayenne, margarine and egg in a blender or food processor. Pulse until the mixture resembles fine bread-crumbs, which will quickly come together to form a ball of dough. As soon as this happens, remove the pastry from the bowl, wrap it in clingfilm (plastic wrap) and chill while you make the filling.
- Heat the oil in a saucepan. Add the onion, with the peppers and herbs, and cook gently for 10 minutes. Stir in the courgettes (zuc-chini) and garlic and simmer for another 10 minutes until the vegeta-bles are soft but not browned. Season the mixture with salt and pepper. Spoon into a bowl and leave to cool while you roll out the pastry.
- Roll the pastry out on a clean surface dusted with flour until it is big enough to cut out the circles to line your tart or muffin tins. Keep the rolling pin and your hands dusted with flour as well. Cut out as many circles as possible from the dough, gather the pastry trimmings to-gether and roll out again to cut a few more circles. Place the pastry in the lined tins and press down gently.
- Stir the yogurt and eggs together in a small bowl, then combine them with the onion mixture. Spoon the filling into each pastry case and sprinkle lightly with cayenne.
- Bake the tarts for 35 minutes or until the pastry is golden and the fill-ing is just firm in the centre. Leave the tarts to cool in the tins, then lift them out carefully, remove the parchment circles and serve warm with a garnish of fresh herbs, salad leaves or edible flowers.

Mushroom and Oregano Pancakes Serves 4

The pancakes used in this delectable dish aren't the type you flip and roll, but rather are Scotch pancakes otherwise known as drop scones. These need to be eaten fresh from the oven for the best results. Keep the cooked pancakes warm and moist in a clean tea towel or napkin until you need them for the final part of the recipe.

- 200g/7oz/1¾ cups of wheat-free flour*
- 2 tsp wheat-free baking powder*
- a pinch each of salt, freshly ground black pepper and cayenne pepper
- 1 tbsp caster (superfine) sugar
- 1 large egg, beaten
- 300ml/½ pint/1¼ cups virtually fat-free milk
- 2 large spring/(scallions) or salad onions, trimmed and very finely sliced
- oil for greasing pan

  * These ingredients should be gluten free for Coeliacs.

For the topping
- 500g/1lb/6 cups of peeled or wiped, trimmed and chopped cultivated mushrooms
- 2 tbsp olive oil
- 20g/³/₄oz/³/₄ cup fresh oregano leaves
- 2 tbsp dry sherry, Madeira or Marsala
- freshly grated nutmeg
- 225g/8oz/1 cup of virtually fat-free fromage frais
- 30g/1oz/1 cup chopped fresh coriander (cilantrol) leaves

- Stir the flour and baking powder with the salt, pepper and cayenne into a bowl. Stir in the sugar and make a well in the centre. Add the egg and milk to the well and stir, gradually incorporating the surrounding flour until you have a smooth batter. Mix in the onions.
- Preheat a griddle or large frying pan (skillet) over high heat and then spray, brush or drizzle with a little oil. Drop tablespoons of the batter on to the surface of the pan. Leave them until they bubble. When the bubbles begin to burst, turn them over with an oiled palette knife and cook until they are golden. Keep hot while you cook the rest of the batter, making 12 pancakes in all.
- Heat the olive oil in a non-stick frying pan (skillet) and add the mushrooms and oregano leaves. Fry over moderate heat for 4–5 minutes. When the mushrooms are soft, stir in the sherry and season with salt, pepper and nutmeg. Shake the pan to coat the mushrooms evenly, then remove from the heat.
- Arrange the pancakes in a line on a warm dish and spoon the mushrooms down the centre. Spoon a line of fromage frais down the centre of the mushrooms, sprinkle with chopped coriander (cilantro) and serve immediately, with a selection of salads, if you like.

Note: This is a delicious starter for 6. Give them two pancakes each, sprinkled with mushrooms and topped with a dollop of fromage frais and a scattering of coriander (cilantro).

Perfect Pizza Serves 4

For years, I was unable to go out with friends for a pizza because they are so wheat and dairy laden! Therefore, I developed a pizza of my own and can now have pizza and wine at home with friends instead.

- 400g/14oz/3½ cups wheat-free flour*, plus extra for dusting and kneading
- ½ tsp salt
- 1 tsp caster (superfine) sugar
- 15g/½oz/1 tbsp easy bake yeast or fast-action dried yeast*
- 300ml/10fl oz/1¼ cups tepid water
- olive oil, for greasing

For the topping
- 1 x 425g/15oz/2 can chopped tomatoes
- 2 tbsp tomato purée (paste)
- chilli sauce* to taste
- 20g/¾oz/¾ cup fresh basil leaves, shredded
- salt and freshly ground black pepper
- stoned black olives
- olive oil, for drizzling
- 115g/4oz reduced fat mozzarella cheese, coarsely grated (or other half-fat hard cheese, goat's, sheep's or vegetarian cheese)
- 2 large non-stick baking sheets

    * These ingredients contain gluten. Coeliacs please substitute them.

- Preheat the oven to 200°C/400°F/Gas mark 6.
- Sift the flour and salt together in a big bowl. Stir in the sugar and yeast. Beat in the water with a wooden spoon and bring the dough together into a ball. You may need to add a little more warm water; different flours absorb varying amounts.
- Put the dough on a floured board and knead with floured hands for 6–10 minutes or until it is smooth. Spray a large bowl with a little olive oil, put the pizza dough into it and cover with a plate or another bowl. Leave the bowl in a warm, draught-free place until the dough has doubled in bulk. This will take 1–2 hours, depending on the temperature of your room.
- Meanwhile you can make the topping. Drain the tomatoes and tip them into a bowl. Stir in the tomato purée (paste), chilli sauce and basil leaves. Season with salt and pepper.
- Place the pizza dough on a floured board and flatten it with a rolling pin. Using a knife, divide it into four equal portions. Roll out each portion on a floured board into a thin 20 cm/8 in circle.
- Place two pizza bases on each baking sheet. Press the dough on each pizza gently outwards with your fingers and pinch up the edges to make a rim and a neat circle. Cover each pizza with the tomato topping, decorate with the olives, drizzle lightly with olive oil and sprinkle with the grated cheese of your choice.
- Bake for 10 minutes or until the crust on each pizza is crisp and golden brown and the cheese on top is bubbling. Carefully slide the pizzas on to hot plates and serve immediately.

Quick Pesto Risotto Serves 2

Desperate for a hot, filling and quick winter's lunch, I used the only four ingredients I had that would produce something instant! The result was so delicious that we now eat it regularly.

- 3 handfuls Italian risotto rice
- 1 x 295g/10½oz/can condensed consommé
- 1 tsp vegetable stock (bouillon) powder
- 4 tsp good quality pesto, preferably organic

- Put the rice in a saucepan with the consommé. Fill the consommé can with water and pour that into the pan. Season with the stock (bouillon) powder and bring to the boil over moderate heat. Stir from time to time and add extra water if the rice becomes dry before it is cooked through. When all the liquid has been absorbed and the rice is cooked through but still moist, stir in the pesto. Serve immediately, on warm plates.

Note: For a vegetarian version of this risotto, use strong vegetable stock instead of the diluted consommé.

Sweet Pepper Pasta Serves 3

This grilled (broiled) pepper sauce makes a delicious alternative to tomato sauce and can be served with any style of pasta from tagliatelle to penne.

- 4 large sweet red peppers, tops cut off and halved, stalk, seeds and pith removed
- 1 tbsp olive oil, plus extra, for brushing peppers
- 1 large onion, trimmed, peeled and chopped
- 1 tsp dried mixed herbs
- 2 cloves garlic, peeled and crushed
- 1 medium fresh chilli of medium strength, halved, deseeded and chopped
- 1 tbsp red wine vinegar
- salt and freshly ground black pepper
- 340g/12oz wheat-free pasta
- 600ml/1 pint/2½ cups of hot water
- a handful of fresh basil leaves, shredded

- Cut off the tops from the peppers and chop the usable pieces roughly. Cut the peppers in half and scoop out the seeds and set the halves aside. Heat the oil in a saucepan. Add the oil and the onions and the chopped pepper pieces. Cook over moderate heat until softened.
- Meanwhile, brush the pepper halves with a little extra oil and then grill (broil) until they have softened and blistered in patches. Peel off the skins and discard them. Chop up the grilled (broiled) peppers and add them to the onion mixture with the mixed herbs, garlic, chilli and vinegar. Season with salt and pepper and stir in the hot water. Cook over moderate heat for about 20 minutes. Leave the sauce to cool and then transfer half of it to a blender or food processor and whizz until smooth. Stir the smooth sauce back into the saucepan and mix it with the chunky sauce with a wooden spoon. Reheat the sauce and adjust the seasoning to taste.
- Cook the pasta in boiling water according to the instructions on the packet. Drain it thoroughly, tip it into a bowl and pour the sauce over. Toss to mix, sprinkle with the shredded basil and serve with a mixed salad, if you like.

Red Onion Clafoutis Serves 4

This is just like a quiche without the pastry! It makes a very good lunch. You can use ordinary onions if red ones are not available, or too expensive.

- 300ml/10fl oz/1¼ cups virtually fat-free milk
- 3 tbsp skimmed milk powder
- 6 tbsp low-fat natural (plain) live yogurt
- 1 medium whole egg, plus 3 whites
- 1 tbsp finely chopped fresh rosemary, tarragon or thyme
- 100g/3½oz/scant 1 cup wheat-free flour
- 4 tbsp grated Parmesan cheese, half-fat hard cheese or vegetarian equivalent

For the topping
- 2 large red onions, trimmed, peeled, halved and finely sliced
- 200ml/7fl oz/generous ¾ cup vegetable stock (bouillon), preferably home-made
- 125ml/4fl oz/½ cup white wine
- salt and freshly ground black pepper
- 23 cm/9 in quiche dish or shallow baking dish

- Preheat the oven to 200°C/400°F/Gas mark 6.
- Put the onions in a saucepan with the stock (bouillon) and bring to the boil. Reduce the heat and simmer until all the liquid has evaporated. Pour in the wine, add salt and pepper to taste, and cook until the onions are soft and the wine has evaporated.
- Meanwhile pour the milk into a bowl and whisk in the milk powder, yogurt, egg and egg whites until smooth. Add the herbs, then whisk in the flour and 3 tablespoons of the cheese.
- Pour the batter into the quiche dish, scatter the onions over the surface, then sprinkle remaining cheese on top. Bake in the centre of the oven for about 30 minutes or until well-risen and golden brown. Serve immediately with a mixed green salad or lightly cooked vegetables.

Spinach stuffed Baked Potatoes Serves 2

Perfect for a cold winter's day, potatoes are warming, filling and healthy. You can make these the day before you plan to serve them. When cool, cover and chill them. Reheat the potatoes in a hot oven or in the microwave before serving. Sweet potatoes can be cooked in exactly the same way, and make a delicious change.

- 2 large baking potatoes
- 115g/4oz/½ cup thawed, frozen chopped spinach
- salt and freshly ground black pepper
- freshly grated nutmeg
- 1 tbsp pine nuts, lightly grilled (broiled) until golden
- 4 tbsp coarsely grated Parmesan, half-fat cheese or the vegetarian equivalent
- cayenne pepper

- Preheat the oven to 200°C/400°F/Gas mark 6.
- Bake the potatoes for 1¼ hours, until they are tender. Meanwhile, drain the spinach in a sieve, pressing out all the excess liquid with a spoon. Carefully transfer to a pad of layered kitchen paper towels to dry completely.
- When the baked potatoes are cool enough to handle, cut them in half and scoop out all the flesh being careful not to damage the skins. Put the flesh into a bowl and mix with the spinach, salt, pepper and nutmeg. Add three-quarters of the pine nuts and 3 tablespoons of the cheese. Mix well, then spoon the mixture back into the potato skins and reshape them.
- Place the stuffed potatoes on to a baking sheet. Sprinkle them with the remaining nuts and cheese and a little cayenne. Bake for about 15 minutes or until the potatoes are very hot and the cheese has melted.

Vegetable Lasagne Serves 6

This is a wonderfully versatile dish. You can use any fresh or frozen vegetables you like or that you have lurking around the refrigerator. Lasagne sheets that are wheat-free are available by mail order (see page 226) or from your local health food store. The variety used below is made from corn.

- 1 tbsp olive oil
- 4 tbsp chopped celery
- 1 large onion, peeled, trimmed and finely chopped
- 8 handfuls finely chopped fresh or frozen vegetables, such as carrots, cauliflower, mushrooms, courgettes (zucchini), broccoli, peppers, beans
- 3 cloves garlic, peeled and crushed
- 1 x 600ml/20fl oz/carton Italian-style fresh tomato soup
- 1 heaped tbsp tomato purée (paste)
- 2 tsp dried mixed herbs
- salt and freshly ground black pepper
- chilli sauce,* to taste
- sugar, to taste
- Orgran instant wheat-free lasagne sheets
- 225g/8oz/1 cup virtually fat-free cottage cheese
- 500g/1lb/2 cups of virtually fat-free fromage frais
- 115g/4oz/1 cup coarsely grated half-fat hard cheese or vegetarian equivalent
- cayenne pepper
- a 30 cm/12 in oblong or oval deep-sided baking dish

  * Coeliacs please replace chilli sauce with a gluten free brand.

- Preheat the oven to 200°C/400°F/Gas mark 6.
- Heat the oil in a large saucepan and cook the celery and onions over moderate heat for about 3 minutes, until slightly softened. Stir in all the other vegetables, with the garlic. Cook until they are slightly softened. Stir in the tomato soup, tomato purée (paste), mixed herbs. Season with salt and pepper and add the chilli sauce and sugar. Cook for a further 5 minutes, then adjust the seasoning.
- Cover the base of the dish with a layer of lasagne sheets. Pour over half the sauce. Cover the sauce with another layer of lasagne sheets, then the remaining sauce.
- In a separate bowl mix the cottage cheese with the fromage frais and hard cheese. Season to taste with salt and pepper. Spread this over the top of the lasagne and sprinkle with cayenne pepper. Bake in the oven for 40 minutes or until the lasagne is cooked through and the top is golden and bubbling. Leave to stand for 5 minutes, so that the layers settle, then serve, accompanied by a green salad with fresh herbs.

Wild Mushroom and Tarragon Tart Serves 6 as a starter,
and 4 as a main course

As dried wild mushrooms are expensive, I mix them with cheaper culti-
vated varieties, but you can use any mushrooms with a good flavour.

- 200g/7oz/1¾ cups wheat-free flour
- 2 tsp mild Dijon mustard
- salt and freshly ground black pepper
- cayenne pepper
- 100g/3½oz/generous ½ cup vegetable margarine
- 1 large egg

For the filling
- 2 tbsp olive oil
- 1 red onion, peeled, trimmed and finely chopped
- 2 pinches of herbes de Provence (mixed herbs)
- 40g/1½oz/2 cups mixed dried wild mushrooms
- 350g/12½oz/4½ cups chopped cultivated mushrooms, trimmed, cleaned (peeled if necessary),
- freshly grated nutmeg
- 4 tbsp dry sherry, Madeira or Marsala
- 370g/13oz/generous 1½ cups natural (plain) Greek-style yogurt or half-fat crème fraiche
- 2 large eggs
- fresh herbs or salad leaves to decorate
- 1 x 23 cm/9 in loose-bottomed, fluted tart tin or quiche dish
- ceramic balls or baking beans

- Preheat the oven to 200°C/400°F/Gas mark 6.
- Put the flour, mustard, salt, pepper , cayenne, margarine and egg in a food processor. Pulse until the mixture resembles fine breadcrumbs, which will quickly come together to form a dough. Wrap the dough in clingfilm (plastic wrap) and chill it while you make the filling.
- Heat half the oil in a large frying pan. Add the onions and herbs and fry for 2–3 minutes. Add the remaining oil, stir in the wild and culti-vated mushrooms, and season with salt, pepper and nutmeg. Cook gently for 3–4 minutes, or until all the oil has been absorbed and the mushrooms are starting to stick to the pan. Pour in the sherry. Cook over low heat until the onions are soft and transparent; do not let them brown. Leave the mixture to cool, then adjust the seasoning to taste.
- Line the loose-bottomed tart tin or quiche dish with a circle of baking parchment. Roll out the pastry on a lightly floured surface and line the prepared tart tin. Press the pastry into the fluted edges and then level the top off with a sharp knife.
- Line the pastry with a circle of baking parchment and weight it down with ceramic balls or baking beans. Bake the pastry blind for 20 minutes, then let it cool before removing the paper and beans. Leave the oven on.
- Beat the yogurt and eggs in a bowl, then stir in the mushroom mix-ture. Pour the mixture into the pastry case and return it to the oven to bake for about 20 minutes or until the filling has set and is golden and firm.
- Serve the tart warm, in slices, with a garnish of fresh herbs or salad leaves.

Desserts and Cakes

Baked Vanilla Fruits Serves 6

You can use a medley of seasonal fruits or simply your favourites. The most successful fruits are pears, apples, pineapple, strawberries, plums, apricots, peaches, nectarines, figs, passion fruit and mangoes.

Choose ripe and fresh-looking fruits to suit your budget and style of menu. For example:

- 2 large pears, peeled, quartered, core and pips removed
- 1 small pineapple, topped and tailed, peeled, halved, inner core removed and cut into 6 wedges
- 3 peaches, wiped clean, halved and stoned
- Plenty of large strawberries, hulled and wiped clean
- 3 plums, wiped clean, halved and stoned
- 500g/1lb 1oz/2 cups fromage frais, to serve

For the syrup
- 1 tbsp caster (superfine) sugar
- 6 tbsp water
- 1 tbsp white rum
- 1/2 tbsp pure vanilla extract

- Preheat the oven to 200°C/400°F/Gas mark 6.
- Make the syrup first. Put the sugar and water into a saucepan and bring it to the boil over moderate heat. Boil for 1 minute then remove the syrup from the heat and stir in the rum and vanilla extract. Set the syrup aside to absorb the flavours and cool down.
- Prepare all the fruit and place it in a big baking tin, grouping the fruits attractively. Drizzle over the syrup and bake for about 10 minutes or until the fruits have softened slightly and are lightly browned at the edges.
- Serve immediately, before the fruits collapse. Accompany the dish with a bowl of chilled fromage frais.

Lemon Curd Roulade Serves 10

This roulade is quick and easy to make and is delicious with afternoon tea for a special occasion. As a summer pudding, serve the roulade with a bowl of fresh raspberries or strawberries. The ideal winter accompaniment would be thinly sliced sweet oranges mixed with some orange flower water and orange liqueur, then chilled.

- 4 large egg whites
- 115g/4oz/½ cup caster (superfine) sugar, plus extra for dusting
- 75g/2½oz/generous ½ cup of wheat-free flour
- grated zest of 1 orange
- 3 tsps fresh orange juice

For the lemon curd filling
- 2 tbsp cornflour (cornstarch)
- 55g/2oz/¼ cup caster (superfine) sugar
- grated zest of 1 lemon and 6 tbsp fresh lemon juice
- 185ml/6fl oz/¾ cup water
- 2 large egg yolks
- 28 x 35 cm/11 x 14 in Swiss roll tin (jelly roll pan)

- Preheat the oven to 150°C/300°F/Gas mark 2. Line the tin with baking parchment or greaseproof (wax) paper.
- Beat the egg whites in a large bowl with an electric mixer until stiff, then gradually beat in the sugar. Fold in the flour and then the orange rind and the juice. Spread the mixture lightly in the prepared tin taking it into all the corners. Bake in the centre of the oven for 7–10 minutes until golden and springy to the touch.
- Lay a sheet of baking parchment on a clean surface and dust it lightly with caster (superfine) sugar. Remove the cooked roulade from the oven and quickly loosen the edges of the cake so that it comes away from the paper. Immediately invert the roulade on the sugared parchment and pull off the lining paper. Roll the lining paper into a sausage shape. Place this on the roulade so that you can roll the cake around it, as though it were a filling. Leave the roulade to get cold.
- Make the lemon curd by combining the cornflour (cornstarch) and sugar with the lemon zest, juice and water in a saucepan. Stir constantly over moderate heat until the mixture comes to the boil and thickens. Remove from the heat and quickly beat in the egg yolks until the mixture is smooth. Cover with baking parchment or greaseproof (waxed) paper and leave to cool at room temperature.
- When you are ready to fill the roulade beat the lemon curd lightly. Carefully unroll the roulade and discard the paper. Spread the lemon curd evenly all over the inside of the cake, roll it back up again and slide it on to a serving dish. Sprinkle with a little extra caster (superfine) sugar and serve.

Strawberry and Raspberry Meringues Serves 6

This is my emergency pudding for unexpected guests, or an instant dessert when all is chaos around me! If fresh strawberries and raspberries are not available, use frozen ones. Tip them into a sieve and use them when they are just thawed.

- 6 ready-made meringue nests or baskets
- 24 (or more) fresh, ripe strawberries, wiped clean, hulled and quartered or halved, depending on size plus 6 whole strawberries to decorate
- 1 x 425g/15oz/can strawberries in fruit juice
- 225g/8oz/2 cups ripe, fresh raspberries
- 2 tsp rosewater
- 6 tiny sprigs of fresh mint, to decorate
- virtually fat-free fromage frais or low-fat dairy or soya ice cream

- Place each meringue on a serving plate and fill them with the prepared fresh strawberries. Drain the canned strawberries reserving the juice. Put the fresh raspberries in a blender or food processor and add the canned strawberries, with two–thirds of the juice. Blend to a purée. Scrape this into a sieve set over a bowl. Using a wooden spoon press the purée through the sieve. Discard the seeds that remain behind.
- Stir the rosewater into the sauce and add extra fruit juice if needed to give a thick pouring consistency. The meringues are very sweet, so you will not need sugar in the sauce.
- Pour the sauce over each meringue, decorate each portion with a fresh strawberry and a little sprig of mint and serve with fromage frais or ice cream.

Chocolate Amaretti Tiramisu Serves 6–8

This pudding is rather less wicked than the original but still tastes delicious and chocolatey.

- 150g/5½oz/2 cups wheat-free ratafias (dessert macaroons) crumbled up into very small pieces
- 1 tbsp white rum mixed with 1 tbsp good quality instant coffee dissolved in 1 tbsp boiling water
- 1 x 11g/½oz/sachet gelatine (or vegetarian equivalent) dissolved with 1 tablespoon of good quality instant coffee and 125ml/4½fl oz/½ cup of boiling water
- 200g/7oz/7 squares good quality dark (bittersweet) chocolate, broken up
- 1 tablespoon brandy
- 2 small eggs, separated
- 500g/1lb 2oz/2 cups virtually fat-free fromage frais
- 250g/9oz/1 cup half-fat crème fraiche
- Cocoa powder to dust

- Fill the base of a glass bowl with the crumbled ratafias (dessert macaroons) and sprinkle them with all of the rum and coffee mixture. Prepare the gelatine (or the vegetarian equivalent).
- Melt the chocolate in a non-stick pan over very low heat with the tablespoon of brandy, stirring occasionally.
- Remove the pan of chocolate from the heat and stir in the 2 egg yolks until smooth. Transfer the chocolate mixture into a bowl and stir in the fromage frais.
- When the gelatine has cooled down to lukewarm it will be ready to use. Vigorously stir the dissolved gelatine and then stir it into the chocolate mixture, until it is evenly blended.
- Now whisk the egg whites in a clean bowl until they form soft peaks and then fold them with a metal spoon into the chocolate mixture.
- Spoon the chocolate over the ratafias (dessert macaroons) and then leave to set in the refrigerator for 3–4 hours or until needed.
- Cover the chocolate with all the crème fraiche and then sift the cocoa over the top.
- Keep the Tiramisu covered and chilled until needed.

Lime Angel Cake Serves 10

This ultra-light cake is perfect for either afternoon tea or as a pudding, when it can be served with one bowl of fresh fruit salad and another of virtually fat-free fromage frais.

- 45g/1½oz/6 tbsp cornflour (cornstarch)
- 45g/1½oz/6 tbsp wheat-free flour
- 8 medium egg whites
- 225g/8oz/1 cup caster (superfine) sugar, plus extra for serving
- grated zest 1 lime
- 1 tbsp of lime juice

To make as a cake
- 5 tbsp icing (confectioners') sugar and 1 extra tbsp lime juice

To make as a pudding
- 3 large, ripe, kiwi fruit, peeled and thinly sliced
- fruit salad or raspberry purée and virtually fat-free fromage frais
- an ungreased angel cake tin or 20 cm/8 in non-stick cake tin

- Preheat the oven to 150°C/300°F/Gas mark 2.
- Sift both flours on to a sheet of greaseproof (wax) paper. Whisk the egg whites in a large bowl until very stiff. Gradually add the sugar, lime zest and lime juice whisking until thick and glossy.
- Gently fold in the flour mixture with a metal spoon. Spoon the cake mixture into the tin and gently level the surface. Bake for about 40 minutes, until the sponge springs back when gently pressed.
- Leave the cake in the tin to cool. Sprinkle a piece of greaseproof paper with the extra caster (superfine) sugar. Then, with the help of a knife, ease the cake out of the tin, invert it on to the paper, then turn it on to a serving plate so that the sugared surface is uppermost.
- For a cake: Make an icing by mixing the icing (confectioner's) sugar with enough lime juice to make a dropping consistency. Drizzle it all over the top of the cake. Keep the cake at room temperature and eat on the day of making.
- For a pudding: Decorate the cake with rows of sliced kiwi fruit. Keep in a cool place and eat on the day of making. Serve with either a fresh exotic fruit salad or a freshly made raspberry purée. Accompany with virtually fat-free fromage frais.

Fruit Cake Serves 12

Dried fruit is a concentrated source of essential minerals, including iron. The sweetness of dried fruit comes from the natural sugar or fructose it contains, so this is a real treat for afternoon tea with the family. It is also perfect to take on a picnic or even as part of a packed lunch for work.

- 130g/4½oz/scant 1 cup of pitted dates, chopped
- 200g/7oz/1 cup ready-to-eat, pitted prunes, chopped
- grated zest of 1 orange
- 250ml/8fl oz/1 cup unsweetened orange juice
- 2 heaped tbsp treacle (molasses)
- 225g/8oz/2 cups wheat-free flour*
- 2 tsp mixed spice* (pie spice)
- 2 tsp cinnamon
- 2 tsp wheat-free baking powder*
- 350g/12½oz/2½ cups mixed dried fruits
- 75g/2½oz/generous ½ cup dried cherries or cranberries
- 3 tbsp brandy
- 3 large egg whites
- 1 tbsp reduced-sugar smooth apricot jam (jelly)
- 20 cm/8 in round, loose-bottomed non-stick cake tin
    * Coeliacs please use gluten free products.

- Preheat the oven to 180°C/350°F/Gas mark 4. Lightly grease the cake tin and line it with baking parchment.
- Combine the dates, prunes and orange zest in a saucepan. Pour in the orange juice and bring to the boil. Reduce the heat and simmer for 10 minutes or until the fruit is very soft.
- Beat in the orange juice until the mixture becomes a purée, stir in the treacle (molasses) and leave to cool.
- Meanwhile, sift the flour, spices and baking powder into a big bowl. Stir in all the mixed dried fruits and dried cherries with the brandy and make a well in the centre.
- In a clean bowl, beat the egg whites until stiff. Spoon the date mixture into the well in the flour and fruit mixture and mix well, gradually incorporating the surrounding flour mixture. Using a metal spoon gently fold in the egg whites then transfer the cake mixture to the prepared tin. Gently level the surface and cover the top of the tin loosely with foil or baking parchment. Bake for 45 minutes, then remove the foil or parchment and bake for 30 minutes more or until a skewer, inserted in the cake, comes out clean.
- Take the cake out of the oven, brush the top with apricot jam (jelly) and let it cool in the tin. When the cake is cold, take it out of the tin and peel off the lining paper. Wrap the cake in foil and store it in an airtight container for 24 hours before eating.

Pear and Cinnamon Slice Serves 8

Just occasionally, when all the family are around at the weekend, I yearn for something sweet. So, as a special treat, I break out and indulge in a small slice of this delicious cake with a steaming cup of espresso. This also makes a yummy winter pudding for special occasions. Serve it just warm, with a bowl of virtually fat-free fromage frais.

- 1 x 425g/15oz/can pear halves in fruit juice
- 285g/10oz/1¼ cups of caster (superfine) sugar
- 1 tbsp ground cinnamon
- 2 large eggs
- 200ml/7floz/generous ¾ cup sunflower oil, plus extra for greasing
- 1 tsp pure vanilla extract
- a pinch of salt
- 240g/8oz/2 cups of wheat-free flour*
- ½ tsp bicarbonate of soda (baking soda)
- 20 cm/8 in round, loose-bottomed non-stick cake tin
  * Coeliacs, please use gluten free brand.

- Preheat the oven to 180°C/350°F/Gas mark 4. Grease the tin very lightly with oil, then line the base with a circle of baking parchment.
- Drain the pears, reserving the juice for another recipe. Slice each pear half into three and leave them to dry in the sieve for 5 minutes. Now place the pears on several layers of kitchen paper towels, cover with a few more layers of paper towels and pat lightly to absorb any remaining moisture. Leave the pears until needed.
- Mix the sugar, cinnamon, eggs and sunflower oil in a bowl. Add the vanilla extract and salt and beat with an electric mixer for 3–4 minutes until well mixed. Sift the flour with the bicarbonate of soda (baking soda) and fold into the egg mixture.
- Fold in the pears, which will loosen the mixture if it is a little dry, then scrape the mixture into the prepared tin. Level the surface and bake the cake for about 1¼ hours or until the cake is firm and springy to the touch.
- Leave the cake in the tin until it is cold, then carefully turn it out on to a serving plate. Cut into 8 slices and do not be tempted to have more than one slice!!

Cinnamon and Oat Crispies Makes 16

Crisp and crunchy cookies are a special treat for all the family. You can adapt the flavours to suit different occasions. Mixed spice (pie spice) or ground ginger instead of cinnamon work extremely well.

- 225g/8oz/2½ cups porridge oats* or oatmeal*
- 75g/2½oz/⅓ cup light or dark muscovado sugar, all lumps removed
- 2 tsp ground cinnamon
- 1 large egg
- 4 tbsp sunflower oil
- 2 tbsp golden syrup (light corn syrup)
- 2 non-stick baking sheets

   * Even though these ingredients contain gluten, some Coeliacs can eat small amounts of oats and oatmeal and so will be able to make this recipe.

- Preheat the oven to 190°C/375°F/Gas mark 5.
- Put the oats, sugar and cinnamon into a bowl. Stir in the egg, oil and syrup. Leave to stand for about 15 minutes.
- Use a dessertspoon to place dollops of the mixture, about 2.5 cm/1 in apart, on both the baking sheets. Using clean hands mould them into round shapes.
- Bake the crispies for 10–12 minutes or until golden brown. Let them cool for 5 minutes before lifting them on to wire racks with a palette knife. Leave until cold.
- Store in an airtight container if you have any left!

Useful Information and Addresses

Information

Antoinette Savill has a website with news, helpful hints and recipes for 'wheat watchers'. The site also includes reviews of her other books, plus a credit card hotline for purchasing books and gluten or wheat-free products.

Website: www.wheatwatchers.com

Dawn Hamilton and her team of qualified nutritionists are available for personal nutritional consultations. This can be conducted face-to-face, by telephone or via the Internet. Dawn is also available for public speaking engagements and training seminars in health and well-being.

Dawn Hamilton and Associates
PO BOX 14035
London
N10 2WB
Telephone: +44 (0)20 8883 2408
Website: www.DawnHamilton.com
Email: info@DawnHamilton.com

Organizations

Institute for Optimum Nutrition
Blades Court
Deodar Road
London SW15 2NU
Telephone: 020 8877 9993

Coeliac Society
PO Box 220
High Wycombe
Buckinghamshire HP11 2HY
Telephone: 01494 437278

The Vegetarian Society
Parkdale
Dunham Road
Altrincham
Cheshire WA14 4QG
Telephone: 01619 280793

Berrydales Publishers
Berrydale House
5 Lawn Road
London NW3 2XS
Telephone: 020 7722 2866
(*The Inside Story* food & health
magazine)

Stockists
United Kingdom

Wellfoods Ltd
(Nationwide delivery of gluten-free
and wheat-free flour and related
products)
Unit 6 Mapplewell Business Park
Mapplewell
Barnsley
S75 6BP

Telephone: 01226 381712
Fax: 01226 381858
Website: www.bake-it.com
Email: wellfoods@bake-it.com

Dietary Specialties
13 Taurus Park
Westbrook
Warrington
WA5 5ZT
Telephone: 07041 544044
Fax: 07041 544055

Orgran Community Foods Limited
(Enquires for stockists of gluten-free
and wheat-free pasta and biscuits
(cookies))
Micross
Brent Terrace
London
NW2 1LT
Telephone: 020 8208 2966
Fax: 020 8208 1551

Doves Farm Foods
(Nationwide delivery of wheat-free
and gluten-free flours and related
products)
Salisbury Road
Hungerford
Berkshire RG17 0RF
Telephone: 01488 684 880
Website: www.dovesfarm.co.uk

Simply Organic Food Company Ltd
(Everything organic – fruit,
vegetables, fish, poultry, meat as
well as groceries, baby food, wines
and wheat or lactose-free products.
All delivered to your home or office
throughout the UK. Open 24 hours
a day, seven days a week.)
Freepost, Units Ab2–A6
New Covent Garden Market
London
SW8 5YY
Telephone: 0845 1000 444
Fax: 020 7622 4447
Website: www.simplyorganic.net
Email: orders@simplyorganic.net

C. Lidgate
(Nationwide delivery of free-range
and organic meats, eggs and
delicatessen)
110 Holland Park Avenue
London W11 4UA
Telephone: 020 7727 8243

Organics Direct Ltd
(Nationwide delivery of baby foods,
wines, beers and all organic
produce)
7 Willow Street
London EC2A 4BH
Telephone: 020 7729 2828
Website: www.organicsdirect.com

The Organic Food Shop
(Nationwide delivery of 4,500 lines,
including teas and cheeses)
45 Broughton St.
Edinburgh EH1 3JU
Telephone: 0131 556 1772

Dr Hauschka Salon
(Fantastic for itchy hay fever eyes
and other allergy-linked skin
problems. Natural & holistic facials,
massage and nail care. Also pure
skin, make up and bath products.)
4 Cheval Place
London SW7 1ES
Telephone: 020 7589 1133
Website:
www.drhauschkasalon.co.uk

Rococo
(Suppliers of sugar-free and dairy-
free chocolate.)
321 Kings Road
London SW3 5EP
Telephone: 020 7352 5857

Higher Nature
(Stockists of FOS powder, an
excellent range of friendly bacteria
supplements and high quality
nutritional supplements.)
Burwash Common
East Sussex
TN19 7LX
Telephone: 01435 882880
Email: sales@higher-nature.co.uk

Selected References

Chapter Two

Dagogo, Jack S et al, 'Robust Leptin Secretory Responses to Dexamethasone in Obese Subjects', *Journal of Clinical Endocrinology and Metabolism*, Vol 82 (10) pp3230–3233, October 1997

Chapter Three

Alfieri MA et al, 'Fiber intake of normal weight, moderately obese and severely obese subjects', *Obesity Research 3*, 541–547, 1995

Burton-Freeman B, 'Dietary fiber and energy regulation', *Journal of Nutrition*, 130, (2S suppl), 272S–275S, 2000

Olesen M and Gudmand-Hoyer E, 'Maldigestion and colonic fermentation of wheat bread in humans and the influence of dietary fat', *The American Journal of Clinical Nutrition*, Vol 66, 62–66, 1997

Chapter Four

Wurtman RJ and Wurtman JJ, 'Brain serotonin, carbohydrate-craving, obesity and depression', *Obesity Research 3*, 477S–480S, 1995

Ismail-Beigi, F, Faraji, B and Reinhold JG, 'Binding of zinc and iron to wheat bread, wheat bran, and their components', *The American Journal of Clinical Nutrition*, Vol 30, 1721–1725, 1977

Chapter Eight

Mori, Trevor A et al, 'Dietary fish as a major component of a weight-loss diet:effect on serum lipids, glucose, and insulin metabolism in overweight hypertensive subjects', *The American Journal of Clinical Nutrition*, Vol 70 (5) 817–825, November 1999

Kris-Etherton, PM et al, 'Polyunsaturated fatty acids in the food chain in the United States', *The American Journal of Clinical Nutrition*, Vol 71, 179–188, January 2000

Other Titles by the Same Authors

The Sensitive Gourmet
by Antoinette Savill
A lavish hardback cook book for the thousands of people suffering from sensitivity to wheat, dairy products and gluten. This book is designed to bring back a pure enjoyment of food and the recipes are smart, modern, international and anything but depriving. It includes menus for special occasions, from a Christmas feast to a summer barbecue.

More from the Sensitive Gourmet
by Antoinette Savill
A glossy sequel which caters for the sweet tooth moments in our lives and those special treats we deserve occasionally. All the recipes are wheat-, dairy- or gluten-free and start with tempting breads and muffins, followed by delicious hot or cold puddings/desserts and ending up with luscious cakes and cookies.

The Gluten, Wheat and Dairy-free Cookbook
by Antoinette Savill
A glamorous slant on virtually fat-free, wheat-free, dairy-free and gluten-free eating. The recipes have been described as 'mouthwatering' and 'positive proof that food intolerances do not mean you have to miss out on delicious treats'. All vegetarian recipes are clearly marked.

Passing Exams: A guide for maximum success and minimum stress
By Dawn Hamilton Ph.D.
There is much more to exam success than just knowing the course material. This book shows you how to revise correctly, manage your time during the exam itself and deal with the inevitable nerves and stress. It contains original techniques that will help you to improve your memory, boost your energy levels and make your brain work better. It will give you the chance to fulfil your potential in any exam situation, whether you are a full-time or part-time student.

Index

Lightning Source UK Ltd.
Milton Keynes UK
14 December 2009

147502UK00001B/127/P